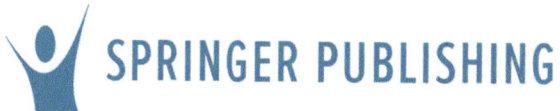

GET THE MOST FROM YOUR BOOK

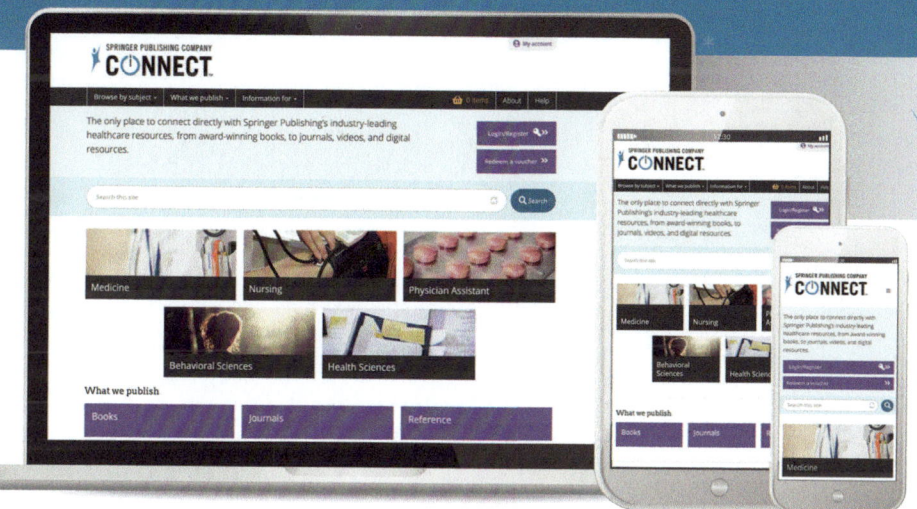

VOUCHER CODE:

3ERBLWTV

Online Access

Your print purchase of *The DNP Project Workbook: A Step-by-Step Process for Success,* Second Edition, includes **online access via Springer Publishing Connect™** to increase accessibility, portability, and searchability.

Insert the code at http://connect.springerpub.com/content/book/978-0-8261-7484-0 or scan the QR code and insert the voucher code today!

Having trouble? Contact our customer service department at **cs@springerpub.com**

Instructor Resource Access for Adopters

Let us do some of the heavy lifting to create an engaging classroom experience with a variety of instructor resources included in most textbooks SUCH AS:

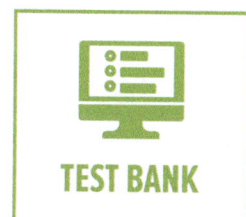

Visit **https://connect.springerpub.com/** and look for the **"Show Supplementary"** button on your **book homepage** to see what is available to instructors! First time using Springer Publishing Connect? Email **textbook@springerpub.com** to create an account and start unlocking valuable resources.

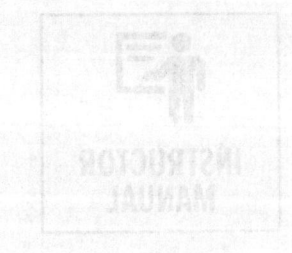

The DNP Project Workbook

Molly Bradshaw, DNP, APRN, FNP-BC, WHNP-BC, CP-C, is the current owner and chief executive officer for her company, DNPmollyB, LLC where she works as a consultant and educator. She maintains a full-time clinical practice at First Choice Immediate Care in Columbia, Kentucky. She completed her undergraduate nursing degrees at Eastern Kentucky University (1998, 2001); got her master's degree at the University of Kentucky (2005); and earned her Doctor of Nursing Practice (DNP) degree at Rutgers, The State University of New Jersey (2016). She is nationally board certified as both a family and a women's health nurse practitioner, as well as a veteran of the United States Navy. In the academic setting she has been a former associate professor, DNP program coordinator, and faculty innovator at Eastern Kentucky University, Richmond, Kentucky. Also, she has been full-time faculty at Rutgers, The State University of New Jersey. Her academic scholarship is rooted in teaching innovation, use of infographics/social media, and the DNP Project. Her published works focus on clinical subjects such as prescribing habits of nurse practitioners and chronic disease management, including hypertension, chronic obstructive pulmonary disease, obesity, and multiple sclerosis. She is engaged in training and content creation for emerging Mobile Integrated Health (MIH) programs and community paramedics.

Tracy R. Vitale, DNP, RNC-OB, C-EFM, NE-BC, has been a nurse for more than 20 years and is currently an associate professor and specialty director of DNP Projects/DNP Project courses at Rutgers, The State University of New Jersey School of Nursing, Newark, New Jersey. She received her baccalaureate degree in nursing from The College of New Jersey (2000), her master's in nursing from the University of Phoenix (2006), and a DNP degree from Rutgers, The State University of New Jersey (2016). Prior to transitioning to academia in 2017, her nursing career included leadership positions in maternal–fetal medicine research, outpatient private maternal–fetal medicine and high-risk obstetrics practice, and labor and delivery/perinatal evaluation and treatment departments. Dr. Vitale sits on the board of directors for the Organization of Nurse Leaders of New Jersey and is actively involved with the research committee. She also serves on the advisory council for the New Jersey Collaborating Center for Nursing, which focuses on nursing workforce issues and is the Region 4 Vice President of Policy and Practice for the New Jersey State Nurses Association. Dr. Vitale also serves as a manuscript reviewer for select journals.

The DNP Project Workbook

A Step-by-Step Process for Success

SECOND EDITION

Molly Bradshaw, DNP, APRN, FNP-BC, WHNP-BC, CP-C

Tracy R. Vitale, DNP, RNC-OB, C-EFM, NE-BC

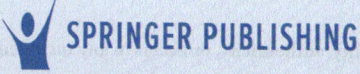

Copyright © 2025 Springer Publishing Company, LLC
All rights reserved.
First Springer Publishing edition 978-0-8261-7432-1 (2020)

No part of this publication may be reproduced, stored in a retrieval system, or transmitted in any form or by any means, electronic, mechanical, photo-copying, recording, or otherwise, without the prior permission of Springer Publishing Company, LLC, or authorization through payment of the appropriate fees to the Copyright Clearance Center, Inc., 222 Rosewood Drive, Danvers, MA 01923, 978-750-8400, fax 978-646-8600, info@copyright.com or at www.copyright.com.

Springer Publishing Company, LLC
902 Carnegie Center/Suite 140, Princeton, NJ 08540
www.springerpub.com
connect.springerpub.com

Acquisitions Editor: Joseph Morita
Production Manager: Kris Parrish
Compositor: diacriTech

ISBN: 978-0-8261-7483-3
ebook ISBN: 978-0-8261-7484-0
DOI: 10.1891/9780826174840

SUPPLEMENTS:

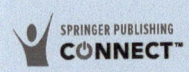 A robust set of instructor resources designed to supplement this text is located at **http://connect.springerpub.com/content/book/978-0-8261-7484-0.**
Qualifying Instructors may request access by emailing **textbook@springerpub.com.**

Instructor Materials:

LMS Common Cartridge (All Instructor Resources) ISBN: 978-0-8261-7489-5
Instructor PowerPoints ISBN: 978-0-8261-7485-7
Instructor and Student Lesson Mapping Tools ISBN: 978-0-8261-4497-3
Mapping to AACN Essentials ISBN: 978-0-8261-7488-8
Transition Guide to the Second Edition ISBN: 978-0-8261-7491-8

Materials available to all purchasers:

Supplementary Editable Activities ISBN: 978-0-8261-7487-1
Rutgers DNP Sample Project ISBN: 978-0-8261-7486-4
Chapter 10 Supplemental DNP Project Documents ISBN: 978-0-8261-4609-0

24 25 26 27 / 5 4 3 2 1

The author and the publisher of this Work have made every effort to use sources believed to be reliable to provide information that is accurate and compatible with the standards generally accepted at the time of publication. Because medical science is continually advancing, our knowledge base continues to expand. Therefore, as new information becomes available, changes in procedures become necessary. We recommend that the reader always consult current research and specific institutional policies before performing any clinical procedure or delivering any medication. The author and publisher shall not be liable for any special, consequential, or exemplary damages resulting, in whole or in part, from the readers' use of, or reliance on, the information contained in this book. The publisher has no responsibility for the persistence or accuracy of URLs for external or third-party Internet websites referred to in this publication and does not guarantee that any content on such websites is, or will remain, accurate or appropriate.

Library of Congress Control Number: 2023054161

Contact sales@springerpub.com to receive discount rates on bulk purchases.

Publisher's Note: New and used products purchased from third-party sellers are not guaranteed for quality, authenticity, or access to any included digital components.

Printed in the United States of America.

In memory of Dr. Sallie Porter, Dr. Tom Christenbery, and Dr. Mary Kamienski, who all gave me some first chances to learn, excel, and succeed. For my grandparents, my family, and my husband Chuck who have always supported me in life, school, work, and faith.

Molly Bradshaw

This text is dedicated to those who have always supported my efforts, encouraged me, and told me I could accomplish anything I put my mind to, especially my parents, Joseph and JoAnne; my husband, Joe; and my children, Joseph and Sophia. I would also like to acknowledge the support of my colleagues, including Lydia, Molly, Sue, and Sharon, for their continued guidance and support. You all have allowed me to achieve more than I could have ever imagined. I hope to inspire others as much as you have done for me. I'd also like to acknowledge those who have literally been by my side throughout this entire nursing journey, including Jack, Harvey, Darius, and Jefferson.

Tracy R. Vitale

Contents

Contributors xi
Foreword   David Anthony Forrester, PhD, RN, ANEF, FAAN   xv
Preface xvii
Resources xxi

1 Ground Zero: Professionalism and Personal Development   1
Editor: Tracy R. Vitale
Contributors: Molly Bradshaw, Margarita David, Krystal Agnew, Angela Clark, Karen O'Connell Schill, Vanessa A. Abacan, and David Coffey

- **Lesson 1.1** Professional Competencies and Communication   4
- **Lesson 1.2** Writing a Professional Bio and Getting Professional Pictures   5
- **Lesson 1.3** Résumé Versus Curriculum Vitae   9
- **Lesson 1.4** Assessment of Personal Learning and Leadership Style   14
- **Lesson 1.5** Developing Basic Technology Skills for the DNP Project   16
- **Lesson 1.6** Developing Writing Skills   18
- **Lesson 1.7** Time Management Strategies   20

2 Understanding the DNP Degree and DNP Project   23
Editors: Brenda Douglass and Sharon Stager
Contributors: Molly Bradshaw, Tracy R. Vitale, Rachel Risner, Sallie Porter, Melissa deCardi Hladek, Deborah Busch, Lisa Grubb, Kimberly McIltrot, Jessica Dean Murphy, Ashly Ninan, Susan Renda, Martha Abshire Saylor, and Brigit VanGraafeiland

- **Lesson 2.1** Why Get a Terminal Degree?   26
- **Lesson 2.2** Nursing Degree Versus Nursing Role   29
- **Lesson 2.3** Understanding the Essentials   32
- **Lesson 2.4** Comparing the DNP and PhD   36
- **Lesson 2.5** Evidence-Based Practice and Quality Improvement   41
- **Lesson 2.6** What Is a DNP Project?   45
- **Lesson 2.7** Design Types of DNP Projects   49
- **Lesson 2.8** DNP Projects Requirements at Your School   53
- **Lesson 2.9** Review of Completed DNP Projects   55
- **Lesson 2.10** The DNP Experience and Practice Hours   59
- **Lesson 2.11** Group DNP Projects   61

3 Identifying Problems and Project Topics 65
Editor: Molly Bradshaw
Contributors: Tracy R. Vitale, Mercedes Echevarria, Patricia Hindin, Jill Cornelison, Sharon Lock, and Maureen Anderson

- **Lesson 3.1** Your Initial Ideas 68
- **Lesson 3.2** Identifying Global and National Problems 70
- **Lesson 3.3** Identifying State and Local Problems 72
- **Lesson 3.4** Problems With the Healthcare System, Information, and Technology 75
- **Lesson 3.5** Cognitive Walkthrough 77
- **Lesson 3.6** Networking to Identify and Discuss Problems 79
- **Lesson 3.7** Organizing Your Findings 82
- **Lesson 3.8** Selecting the Problem and Drafting the Problem Statement 84

4 Developing the DNP Project Background and Context 91
Editor: Molly Bradshaw
Contributors: Tracy R. Vitale and Karen Gilbert

- **Lesson 4.1** Initial Inquiry and Initial Search 93
- **Lesson 4.2** Finding Evidence and Data to Document the Problem 98
- **Lesson 4.3** Strategic Agendas Related to the Problem 100
- **Lesson 4.4** Clinical Guidelines Related to the Problem 102
- **Lesson 4.5** Policies Related to the Problem 104
- **Lesson 4.6** Using the Quadruple Aim to Examine the Problem 107
- **Lesson 4.7** Impact of the Problem on Patients, Families, and Communities: Social Determinants of Health 109
- **Lesson 4.8** Impact of the Problem on Organizations 112
- **Lesson 4.9** Demonstrating the Value of the DNP Project 115
- **Lesson 4.10** Putting It All Together—The DNP Project Outline: Draft #1 118

5 Review of Literature, Evidence Appraisal, and PICO Question Development 123
Editor: Aaron M. Sebach
Contributors: Molly Bradshaw, Tracy R. Vitale, Margaret Dreker, Irina Benenson, and Marilyn Oermann

- **Lesson 5.1** Types of Evidence and Literature Reviews 126
- **Lesson 5.2** Formalizing a PICO Question 131
- **Lesson 5.3** Selecting Appropriate Databases 134
- **Lesson 5.4** Documenting Your Search, Annotation, and Citation Management 139
- **Lesson 5.5** Options for Evidence Appraisal 144
- **Lesson 5.6** Appraisal, Comparison, and Reconciliation of Clinical Practice Guidelines 146
- **Lesson 5.7** Constructing an Evidence Table 149
- **Lesson 5.8** Synthesizing the Evidence 150

6 Assembling the DNP Project Team and Preparing to Lead Change 155
Editor: Tracy R. Vitale
Contributors: Molly Bradshaw, Mercedes Echevarria, and David Anthony Forrester

- **Lesson 6.1** Historic Nursing Leadership to Frame Your Leadership Role 158
- **Lesson 6.2** You Are the Champion of Change 161
- **Lesson 6.3** Why Team Versus Committee? 162
- **Lesson 6.4** DNP Team Roles 164
- **Lesson 6.5** Creating Your DNP Team 170
- **Lesson 6.6** Considerations for Project Feasibility 171

- **Lesson 6.7** Articulating Desired Project Outcomes 175
- **Lesson 6.8** Writing a Purpose Statement 177
- **Lesson 6.9** DNP Project Theory 179
- **Lesson 6.10** Putting It All Together—An Outline 181

7 Project Methodology: Develop, Implement, and Evaluate 185
Editor: Fontaine Sands
Contributors: Molly Bradshaw, Tracy R. Vitale, Debra Bingham, Nancy Owens, and Gina Purdue

- **Lesson 7.1** Perspectives on DNP Project Methods 188
- **Lesson 7.2** Developing Aims and Specific, Measurable, Achievable, Relevant, Time-Bound Objectives 190
- **Lesson 7.3** Think Beyond Education 194
- **Lesson 7.4** Implementation Frameworks and DNP Project Design 196
- **Lesson 7.5** Intervention Population, Inclusion/Exclusion Criteria, and Recruitment 198
- **Lesson 7.6** Collaborative Institutional Training Initiative Training and Ethical Considerations 201
- **Lesson 7.7** Participation Consent 204
- **Lesson 7.8** Evaluation of Outcomes and Process 206
- **Lesson 7.9** Project Data and Plans for Data Analysis 209
- **Lesson 7.10** Timeline, Budget, and Resources 212
- **Lesson 7.11** Anticipated Findings 215
- **Lesson 7.12** Institutional Review Board: Application Considerations 216

8 Strategies to Organize, Disseminate, and Sustain DNP Project Findings 221
Editor: Tracy R. Vitale
Contributors: Molly Bradshaw, Thomas Christenbery, and David G. Campbell-O'Dell

- **Lesson 8.1** Project Management 224
- **Lesson 8.2** Writing the Results and Discussion Sections 226
- **Lesson 8.3** Writing About Impact and Implications 229
- **Lesson 8.4** Completing the Final Academic Paper 231
- **Lesson 8.5** Skills for Oral Presentations 233
- **Lesson 8.6** Strategies for Creating Scholarly Posters 235
- **Lesson 8.7** DNP Project Repositories 239
- **Lesson 8.8** Social Media and Alternative Dissemination 241

9 The DNP Experience 247
Editor: Molly Bradshaw
Contributors: Tracy R. Vitale and Irina Benenson

- **Lesson 9.1** Understanding the DNP Experience Hours 250
- **Lesson 9.2** American Association of Colleges of Nursing Essential Subcompetency Outliers 252
- **Lesson 9.3** Creating a DNP Portfolio 255
- **Lesson 9.4** Honing Your Political Awareness and Engagement 257
- **Lesson 9.5** Developing Business Skills 259
- **Lesson 9.6** Data Visualization 262
- **Lesson 9.7** DNP Engagement in Research and Systematic Reviews 264
- **Lesson 9.8** Developing Your Qualifications as a Nurse Educator 267
- **Lesson 9.9** Safety and Preparedness Skill Development 270

- **Lesson 9.10** Just Culture and the DNP Project 271
- **Lesson 9.11** Inclusion of Interprofessional Interactions 273

10 Finishing Strong: Project Profiles and Empowerment 275
Editor: Jeannie Scruggs Cory
Contributors: Molly Bradshaw, Tracy R. Vitale, Linda Shepard, and Tina C. Switzer

- **Lesson 10.1** DNP Project Profile: Implementing Evidence-Based Messages 277
- **Lesson 10.2** DNP Project Profile: Use of the Institute for Healthcare Improvement Model for Improvement 280
- **Lesson 10.3** DNP Project Profile: Community-Based Projects and Population Health 283
- **Lesson 10.4** DNP Project Profile: Advocacy to Create a Body of Scholarship 286
- **Lesson 10.5** DNP Project Profile: Recovering After Your Topic Changes 289
- **Lesson 10.6** DNP Project Profile: Nursing Leadership and Competency Development 292
- **Lesson 10.7** DNP Project Profile: Program Evaluation—Population Health 295
- **Lesson 10.8** The Approach to "Negative" or "Bad" Results 298
- **Lesson 10.9** Finishing on a Note of Empowerment 300

Appendix: Project Management Resources 303
Index 309

Contributors

CONTRIBUTORS TO THE SECOND EDITION

Vanessa A. Abacan, DNP, APRN, ACCNS-P, RNC-MNN, EBP-C
Student Contributor
Johns Hopkins School of Nursing
Baltimore, Maryland

Krystal Agnew, DNP, APRN, FNP-BC
Student Contributor
Bradley University
Peoria, Illinois

Maureen Anderson, DNP, APN, CRNA
Assistant Professor, Director of Simulation
Division of Advanced Nursing Practice, Rutgers School of Nursing
Rutgers, The State University of New Jersey
New Brunswick, New Jersey

Irina Benenson, DNP, FNP-C, CEN
Associate Professor
Division of Advanced Nursing Practice, Rutgers School of Nursing
Rutgers, The State University of New Jersey
Newark, New Jersey

Molly Bradshaw, DNP, APRN, FNP-BC, WHNP-BC, CP-C
Owner/CEO of DNPmollyB, LLC
Nurse Practitioner
First Choice Immediate Care, Cumberland Family Medical Centers
Columbia, Kentucky

Katherin Brandt, DNP, RN, PHN, CNE, CENP
Student Contributor
Eastern Kentucky University
Richmond, Kentucky;
Interim Dean, Health Science and Nursing Division
Rio Hondo College
Whittier, California

Deborah Busch, DNP, CPNP-BC, IBCLC, CNE, FAANP, FAAN
Associate Professor
John Hopkins School of Nursing
Baltimore, Maryland

David G. Campbell-O'Dell, DNP, APRN, FNP-BC, FAANP
President
Doctors of Nursing Practice, Inc.
Key West, Florida

Angela Clark, DNP, RNC-OB
Student Contributor
Eastern Kentucky University
Richmond, Kentucky;
Assistant Professor
University of Kentucky
Lexington, Kentucky

David Coffey, DNP, APRN, CPNP-PC
Clinical Faculty
Eastern Kentucky University
Richmond, Kentucky

Margarita David, DNP, BA, RN, PCCN, CSN
Director of Programming
Rowan University
Stratford, New Jersey

Mary DiGuilio, DNP, APN, FAANP
Associate Chair of Graduate Nursing/Director of NP Program
Moravian University
Bethlehem, Pennsylvania

Brenda Douglass, DNP, APRN, FNP-C, CDCES, CTTS
Assistant Professor
Johns Hopkins University
Baltimore, Maryland

Mercedes Echevarria, DNP, APN-C
Associate Professor and Assistant Dean for the Doctor of Nursing Practice Program
George Washington University
Washington, DC

Lisa Grubb, DNP, MSN, BSN, RN
Assistant Professor
Johns Hopkins School of Nursing
Baltimore, Maryland

Melissa deCardi Hladek, PhD, CRNP, FNP-BC
Assistant Professor
John Hopkins School of Nursing
Baltimore, Maryland

Kimberly McIltrot, DNP, CPNP, CWOCN, CNE, FAANP, FAAN
Associate Professor
John Hopkins School of Nursing
Baltimore, Maryland

Jessica Dean Murphy, DNP, CRNP, CPNP-AC, CPHON, CNE
Instructor
John Hopkins School of Nursing
Baltimore, Maryland

Ashly Ninan, DNP, APRN, FNP-BC
Performance Improvement Specialist Quality Management
Johns Hopkins Bayview Medical Center
Baltimore, Maryland

Marilyn Oermann, PhD, RN, ANEF, FAAN
Thelma M. Ingles Professor of Nursing
Director of Evaluation and Educational Research
Duke University
Durham, North Carolina

Nancy Owens, DNP, APRN, FNP-C
Associate Professor
Department of Baccalaureate and Graduate Nursing
Eastern Kentucky University
Richmond, Kentucky

Gina Purdue, DNP, RN, CNE
Associate Professor
Department of Baccalaureate and Graduate Nursing
Eastern Kentucky University
Richmond, Kentucky

Susan Renda, DNP, ANP-BC, CDCES, FNAP, FAAN
Associate Professor, Associate Director of DNP Advanced Practice Program
John Hopkins School of Nursing
Baltimore, Maryland

Rachel Risner, PhD, DNP, APRN, C-FNP, CNE
Associate Dean of Academic Affairs
Frontier University
Hyden, Kentucky

Fontaine Sands, DrPH, MSN, RN, CIC
Full Professor, School of Nursing
Eastern Kentucky University
Richmond, Kentucky

Michelle Santoro, DNP, APN, FNP-C
Student Contributor
Rutgers School of Nursing
Newark, New Jersey

Martha Abshire Saylor, PhD, RN
Assistant Professor
Johns Hopkins School of Nursing
Baltimore, Maryland

Karen O'Connell Schill, DNP, APN-C, FNP–BC, ENP-C, CEN, CFRN, NRP
Clinical Assistant Professor
Division of Advanced Nursing Practice, Rutgers School of Nursing
Newark, New Jersey

Jeannie Scruggs Corey, DNP, MSN
Professor, School of Nursing
James Madison University
Harrisonburg, Virginia

Aaron M. Sebach, PhD, DNP, MBA, AGACNP, FNP, CNE, CNEcl, SFHM, FNAP, FAANP
Dean, College of Health Professions and Natural Sciences
Wilmington University
New Castle, Delaware

Linda Shepard, DNP, MBA, BSN, RN, NEA-BC
Student Contributor
James Madison University
Harrisonburg, Virginia

Lori Smith, DNP, APRN, FNP-C
Assistant Professor
Director of the Graduate Nursing Program
Henderson State University
Arkadelphia, Arkansas

Sharon Stager, DNP, APRN, FNP-BC
Associate Professor
Salve Regina University
Newport, Rhode Island

Tina C. Switzer, DNP, RN, CNL
Assistant Professor
School of Nursing
James Madison University
Harrisonburg, Virginia

Brigit VanGraafeiland, DNP, CRNP, CNE, FAAN, FAANP
Associate Professor, Associate Director of DNP Executive Program
Johns Hopkins School of Nursing
Baltimore, Maryland

Tracy R. Vitale, DNP, RNC-OB, C-EFM, NE-BC
Associate Professor
Division of Advanced Nursing Practice, Rutgers School of Nursing
Rutgers, The State University of New Jersey
Newark, New Jersey

CONTRIBUTORS TO THE FIRST EDITION

Tracy Arnold, DNP, RN

Debra Bingham, DrPH, RN, FAAN

Brenda Caudill, DNP, APRN

Thomas Christenbery, PhD, RN, CNE[*]

Jill Cornelison, DNP, RN

Martha De Crisce, DNP, APN, FNP-C

Margaret Dreker, MPA, MLS

David Anthony Forrester, PhD, RN, ANEF, FAAN

Karen Gilbert, MLS, MPH

Patricia Hindin, PhD, CNM, RYT 200

Christine Leithead, DNP, APRN, FNP-C

Sharon Lock, PhD, APRN, FNAP, FAANP

Tarnia Newton, DNP, MSN, FNP-C

Aleksandra Novik, BBA, DNP, APN-C

Sallie Porter, DNP, PhD, APN, RN-BC, CPNP[*]

Lori Smith, DNP, APRN, FNP-C

Grace H. Sun, DNP, APRN, FNP-BC

Angela Wood, DNP, APRN, FNP-C, PPCNP-BC

Margaret Zoellers, DNP, APRN, FNP-BC

---

[*]Deceased.

Foreword

After the success of our first edition of *The DNP Project Workbook: A Step-by-Step Process for Success*, it is a privilege to continue to support students looking to earn their Doctor of Nursing Practice (DNP) degree with the aspirations of leading nursing, healthcare, and society now and into the future.

The DNP degree is a leadership credential in problem-solving. As a DNP-prepared nurse, you will be expected to lead nursing, health policy, and healthcare. In fact, a key tenet of the Institute of Medicine's (IOM's) report, *The Future of Nursing: Leading Change, Advancing Health* (IOM, 2011), is that "Nurses should be full partners, with physicians, and other health professionals, in redesigning healthcare in the United States" (p. 8). This means that as a DNP-prepared nurse, you will be expected to lead interprofessional partnerships and collaborate with stakeholders at every level of the current and future healthcare system, including among nurse generalists, APRNs, and other healthcare providers and policy makers.

According to the American Association of Colleges of Nursing (AACN, 2021), the purpose of designing and implementing a scholarly, evidence-based DNP Project is that it should be an academic experience that allows you to demonstrate competency of the *Essentials*. Achieving these *Essentials* requires you to engage in leadership behaviors and utilize evidence to solve complex problems. The DNP Project experience should help prepare you to lead changes at the highest levels of clinical practice and policy and ultimately improve the overall quality of healthcare (AACN, 2021).

The healthcare environment is rapidly changing and demanding better care for individuals, improved health outcomes for populations, and lower costs for consumers. In this new environment of rapid change and increasing complexity, DNP-prepared nurses are being challenged to lead healthcare systems that offer universal accessibility, coordination across all points of care, and the delivery of high-quality, safe care—and all this at an affordable price. This environment challenges DNP-prepared nurses to understand and embrace collaboration, team-based care, and partnerships and to focus on providing excellence for healthcare consumers in achieving optimal health outcomes (Salmond & Forrester, 2016).

Informed by the historical underpinnings of nursing and advanced practice nursing, this workbook provides DNP students with the strategies to engage in evidence-based practice change and leadership opportunities in which to apply these strategies to the realities of advanced practice nursing. It offers DNP students a clear focus on professional practice, clinical leadership, and policy making. Here, leadership is conceptualized as being concerned with the APRN's ability to influence others by building highly productive teams and identifying and working with stakeholders to reach specific goals to achieve excellence in nursing and healthcare.

This book offers a wealth of strategies that will be tremendously helpful to DNP students in achieving excellence by developing, implementing, evaluating, and disseminating high-quality DNP Projects. Real-world examples and useful exercises are provided. DNP students are challenged to think critically, anticipate and plan, and be strategic in their decision-making in choosing meaningful, feasible project designs and methods. Students are invited to look ahead to the future and ponder the possibilities of a desired future for nursing and healthcare.

This book is an excellent resource for guiding the next generation of DNP-prepared nurses who strive to lead and improve patient-related outcomes. It is my hope that *The DNP Project Workbook: A Step-by-Step Process for Success* will educate, inspire, and empower its readers to lead nursing, health, healthcare, and society into a better, healthier future.

Please enjoy your journey as you proceed with your DNP program of study and carry out your DNP Project.

David Anthony Forrester, PhD, RN, ANEF, FAAN
Professor, Division of Nursing Science, Rutgers University School of Nursing
Clinical Professor, Rutgers University Robert Wood Johnson Medical School
New Brunswick, New Jersey

REFERENCES

American Association of Colleges of Nursing. (2015). *The doctor of nursing practice: Current issues and clarifying recommendations*. Retrieved from https://www.aacnnursing.org/Portals/42/News/White-Papers/DNP-Implementation-TF-Report-8-15.pdf

Institute of Medicine. (2011). *The future of nursing: Leading change, advancing health*. Washington, DC: National Academies Press. Retrieved from http://www.nationalacademies.org/hmd/Reports/2010/The-Future-of-Nursing-Leading-Change-Advancing-Health.aspx

Salmond, S. W., & Forrester, D. A. (2016). Nurses leading change: The time is now! In D. A. Forrester (Ed.), *Nursing's greatest leaders: A history of activism* (pp. 269–286). New York, NY: Springer Publishing Company.

Preface

WHY YOU NEED THIS WORKBOOK

The Doctor of Nursing Practice (DNP) degree requires the completion of a DNP Project. For most students, the thought of this academic requirement is overwhelming at first. The most difficult part is the beginning. You need a place to start. You need a process to follow that creates momentum toward success. We are here to help! Let us be your guide. The purpose of this workbook is to deliver a step-by-step process toward finishing your DNP Project. The lessons engage you in active learning, give you real-world context, and support you with practical tips and advice. The workbook helps you avoid stalemate, minimizes your frustration, and encourages you to think like an innovative problem-solver. Our goal is to help you and your team make meaningful changes in practice that can improve health outcomes for the patients and populations we serve.

THE VISION AND INSPIRATION FOR THIS WORK

The vision for this workbook started with our own DNP experiences. I know now that my experience was typical. I struggled in the beginning. I changed my topic around and couldn't seem to find that perfect question to ask. Faculty used words and phrases that contradicted. For example, one would say "Your research project," and then another would say "No, you are not doing research," which confused me terribly. I could not sort out what was good to know in class versus what I needed to know for creating the project. I felt like certain classmates were ahead of me, that their ideas were so great, and that I was falling behind. It was all overwhelming, to the point of tears. I didn't know how to break down the process of creating the project.

My classmate Tracy R. Vitale also had reservations at the beginning of the process. "Making the decision to even return for a DNP was not easy. Maybe it was the 5-year-old twins, two dogs, and the husband I had at home or trying to figure out how I would balance working full time with returning to school full time. I came to the program having a general idea of the topic I wanted my DNP Project to be about . . . even though I didn't quite know exactly what the actual project would be." The good news is that we all made it. We all graduated. But having a workbook to break down the steps would have been tremendously helpful.

Frustration with the DNP Project process became my motivator. Being a nurse educator in a sprawling BSN–DNP program, I committed to finding out for myself everything to be known about the DNP Project. I was going to make myself an expert and learn to teach the components of project development in a systematic way. My timing coincided with an opportunity to become the director of DNP Projects at my school. What followed next became the basis of what we teach you in this workbook.

First, I created key documents for our department. These documents outlined the minimum requirements for the DNP Project as described by the American Association of Colleges of Nursing (AACN). I made a chart comparing the differences between the DNP and PhD degrees. I rewrote the DNP tool kit for our school and pitched it to the faculty for approval. These revised documents and quick references helped create a more common language to use when discussing the DNP Project. (We are going to share similar documents with you in this workbook.)

Then, with these faculty-approved documents in hand, I started hosting "DNP Project workshops." The workshops were offered outside of classroom time and ahead of courses in which the DNP Project proposal would be written. It gave students an opportunity to learn about the specifics of the project, do exercises to develop their ideas, and get feedback in a group context. Students commented

- "I have a better understanding and foundation of what the DNP Project is and what I need to complete. Having taken this workshop, I no longer feel like a 'deer in headlights.' Despite still feeling apprehensive and anxious about the process, I have a stronger feeling that I can complete this within the time frame allotted."
- "Just the fact that we got an insight on what the project is about and what the steps will be in completing it. I knew nothing about this project and was terrified of it, but after coming to this workshop I feel a bit more comfortable knowing what is expected."

I tracked the attendees over the course of their DNP Projects and found that those who attended the workshops experienced less anxiety and made better overall project progress compared to their peers. As a final step, I began a basic audit of the DNP Projects completed by the graduating class. I used the DNP *Essentials* and the minimum DNP Project requirements outlined by AACN (2015) as a starting point. This process gave me better clarity on what elements need improvement in our program.

Ultimately, the inspiration for this work centers first on you—my student, my colleague. Students in DNP programs are RNs. Therefore, we are already colleagues. As a faculty member or mentor, you are hiring me, engaging me, to help guide you to a higher level of practice. Our commitment to you in return is to make things as simple, manageable, and feasible as possible. If you work hard with us, you will finish strong. But our real driver has to be our patients. They face complex problems and need our help. The DNP degree is about giving you a new skill set to assist your patients. The DNP Project is an opportunity to practice those skills in a real-world context, with the help and guidance of your DNP faculty.

WHAT TO EXPECT FROM THE WORKBOOK

The DNP Project Workbook: A Step-by-Step Process for Success is a collection of individual lessons spanning 10 chapters. Overall, the workbook starts with fundamental, knowledge-based information regarding the DNP Project. It then moves through the development of the DNP team, the feasibility of project ideas, and later through the elements of developing, implementing, evaluating, disseminating, and sustaining the project. Real-world projects are explored in Chapter 10, and tips, advice, and expert commentary are offered throughout.

The lessons are designed to be completed in short intervals. In our experience, DNP students are better able to complete shorter lessons over a given time span. This makes it easier to manage with full-time work, families, and so on. Each lesson gives you some brief background information and then leads you through an active learning exercise. At the end of each lesson, we offer advice for next steps, remind you of key milestones, and recommend additional references and resources. The lessons build on one another as the chapter progresses.

The workbook is designed with usability and flexibility in mind. Open white space is available in each lesson if you prefer to write directly in the workbook. Electronic versions are offered as well; these can be filled out electronically if you need to send a copy to a faculty member. You might need a fresh clean copy to begin a lesson again. There are forms that will help you better document and organize ideas, communicate with stakeholders, and track your progress. Also, we understand that there is variation across DNP programs in terms of the order in which content is taught. Having the lessons broken down individually allows you to complete them in the order that best correlates with the requirements at your school. In addition, the workbook includes useful instructor resources so that the process can be easily implemented into courses—there are PowerPoint slides that summarize content and chapters, and lessons are mapped to the AACN (2021) *Essentials*.

This is a unique product because it is a workbook, not a "textbook" in the traditional sense. It is a platform intended to generate momentum. Our tone and language are purposely nonacademic, conversational, and slightly raw. We want you to feel that we are guiding you and teaching you as mentors. We recognize that this information is not always comprehensive. Rather, it is a place to start. To supplement the context of activities, we refer to outside sources, like the Institute for Healthcare Improvement (IHI). We draw inspiration from outside, nonhealthcare business concepts. We also correlate the content of the lessons with more detailed reading available in the Springer Publishing DNP library. If you find that you need more information, we point out target chapters, specific content, and additional resources that you can further explore.

A LIVING PROCESS

We often refer to the DNP Project process as a "living process." It is organic, growing, and always under development. Why? Because it is a practice-focused doctorate. Practice changes. Practice evolves. As the healthcare system evolves, as patients/populations evolve, as evidence evolves, so must the DNP Project process. The DNP Projects of today should look nothing like the DNP Projects of the future. We must change to meet the needs of the patients and the discipline.

The constant here is the approach we take to solving problems. What is the problem? What has been done so far to address the problem? What resources and evidence do we have to inform solutions? Can we implement a change in practice and measure its impact? Should we continue that practice or abandon it and make new changes? It is the approach to problem-solving that helps us set a standard for "minimum expectations" of a DNP Project. The key milestones lead to addressing a problem in practice.

This is a critical conversation because as a student you will hear faculty talking about "rigor" in the DNP Project process. We talk about this more in the workbook, but for now, embrace the idea of quality. We want you to do quality work that meets a minimum set of expectations based on national standards and the requirements at your school. The minimum expectations ensure a degree of equity among DNP Projects.

"But I want to do a 'good' project," you say? Of course, we want that for you, too. But remember that you are entering a living process. As you complete this work, we ask that you and your faculty be open to new ideas. A "good" project is a completed project that engaged a student in a meaningful learning experience while meeting national and program expectations. There is no such thing as a "perfect" project, unless unicorns also exist.

FINAL THOUGHTS

Together, our experience offers a variety of perspectives as both faculty and former DNP students. We are both still engaged in clinical practice—I am a nurse practitioner and Tracy, my coauthor, is a nurse leader. We represent a DNP spectrum: (a) a large, research-based school of nursing in an urban setting and (b) a smaller regional, online program, catering to rural populations. In this workbook, we present to you a united front of DNP content to serve you so that you can impact your communities, our nation, and the world.

Regardless of the size of your institution, DNP core courses are based on the *Essentials*. The core courses of a DNP curriculum offer opportunities for you to gain new knowledge and skills. This allows you to examine a complex problem through multiple lenses. Each course offers something that can contribute to the DNP Project. The DNP Project will morph as you complete these courses. Do not expect your first ideas to be your final ideas or you will likely be disappointed. Sit back, keep an open mind, and learn something new.

The common thread of problem-solving runs through the fibers of nursing and at our core is a constant in our profession. We are problem-solvers. That is truly what the DNP degree is all about. Keep in mind that this is hard work; it should be—you will graduate with a doctoral degree. We want to help you through this process step-by-step. Hang with us. Just start here, let's work hard, and you will finish strong!

Molly Bradshaw

Resources

All purchasers of this text have access to the following resources at https://connect.springerpub.com/content/book/978-0-8261-7484-0:

- Supplementary Editable Activities
- Rutgers DNP Sample Project
- Supplemental DNP Project Documents to Accompany Chapter 10 Activities

INSTRUCTOR RESOURCES

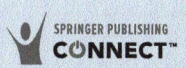 A robust set of instructor resources designed to supplement this text is located at http://connect.springerpub.com/content/book/978-0-8261-7484-0. Qualifying Instructors may request access by emailing textbook@springerpub.com.

- LMS Common Cartridge With All Instructor Resources
- Instructor PowerPoint Presentations
- Instructor and Student Lesson Mapping Tools
- Mapping to AACN Essentials: Core Competencies for Professional Nursing Education
- Transition Guide: First to Second Edition

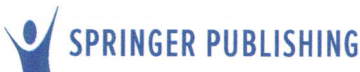

To access supplementary materials, visit https://connect.springerpub.com/978-0-8261-7484-0 and look for the **"Show Additional Resources"** button on the **book homepage**.

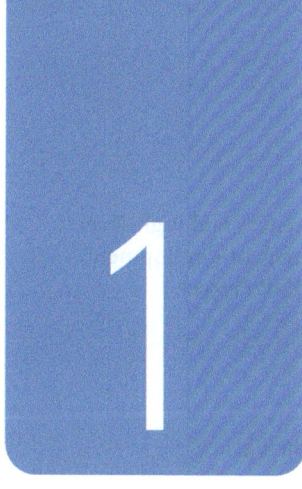

Ground Zero: Professionalism and Personal Development

Editor: Tracy R. Vitale
Contributors: Molly Bradshaw, Margarita David, Krystal Agnew, Angela Clark, Karen O'Connell Schill, Vanessa A. Abacan, and David Coffey

Lessons

Lesson 1.1 Professional Competencies and Communication

Lesson 1.2 Writing a Professional Bio and Getting Professional Pictures

Lesson 1.3 Résumé Versus Curriculum Vitae

Lesson 1.4 Assessment of Personal Learning and Leadership Style

Lesson 1.5 Developing Basic Technology Skills for the DNP Project

Lesson 1.6 Developing Writing Skills

Lesson 1.7 Time Management Strategies

OBJECTIVES

The purpose of this chapter is to help DNP students prepare for professional experiences and high-level academic work. The topics selected have been identified by DNP faculty as key areas of development. Ideally, students should invest time in developing these skills prior to starting their DNP Project.

By the end of this chapter, you will be able to:

- Communicate in a professional manner.
- Present a professional identity in various formats.
- Demonstrate competency in writing, time management, and use of emotional intelligence.

INTRODUCTION

As you start the DNP Program, you may notice that your faculty frequently talk about "competencies." Competency, simply put, means that you have demonstrated an ability to perform a task successfully. In your DNP Program, you will be asked to perform professional tasks that require a sophisticated approach. Your work must be high-level, polished, thoughtful, and intentional. A doctoral student must be competent in key professional skills prior to starting the DNP Project.

The American Association of Colleges of Nursing (2021) have emphasized this point. In their document *The Essentials, Core Competencies for Nursing Education* (2021), they devote an entire domain to the idea. Sub-competencies mention ethical behavior, communication, professional identity, and professional growth. Faculty will ensure that these skills are validated.

The challenge is that everyone may be starting from a different point. Students completing the DNP degree vary in terms of professional and life experience. For example, seasoned nurses may be finishing a post-master's degree. In contrast, other nurses may be new and inexperienced. It may have been a number of years since you have written an academic paper, technology changes, and professional use of social media is mainstream. Therefore, it is important that you consider your own starting point prior to engaging in DNP Project work. Talk with your faculty as you work.

In this chapter, you will be challenged to do a personal inventory. To review the status of your own professional preferences, skills, and appearance. DNP faculty have identified a need for students to improve their professional skills. You will also need to have some of these items ready to present yourself to an agency as a candidate who can lead a project. We will also let you in on some pet peeves and things DNP faculty want students to know.

REFERENCES AND RESOURCES

American Association of Colleges of Nursing. (2021). *The essentials: Core competencies for professional nursing education*. https://www.aacnnursing.org/Education-Resources/AACN-Essentials

MY GOALS FOR DEVELOPING MYSELF PROFESSIONALLY AND AS A LEADER INCLUDE:

LESSON 1.1

PROFESSIONAL COMPETENCIES AND COMMUNICATION

BACKGROUND

In this lesson, we will review the American Association of Colleges of Nursing (AACN) recommendations on professional competency and professional development. Your work on this lesson will prepare you for a conversation with your faculty to further determine how your DNP Project will challenge your professional growth.

We feel it is important to emphasize the importance of communication from the start. To complete a DNP Project, you will have to have multiple conversations with both your faculty and the partnering agency. Professionalism is key. Be polite, be clear, be consistent, and be ready to document your conversation. As the project evolves, it is imperative to keep a record of your communications with your DNP team, mentors, site/content experts, and others.

Here are some professional communication tips that DNP faculty want to emphasize.

- **Keep a communication log.** Document dates when you communicated, topics discussed, and next steps. Keeping this log allows you to establish clear goals and timelines to keep you on track.
- **Consider timing.** If you are asking someone to read your paper and provide constructive feedback, recognize it is unrealistic to expect a return of your paper within 24 to 48 hours. Faculty, editors, and writing centers, among others, are busy. Although your work is certainly important, reading your paper is not their only obligation and other work may be of higher priority. If you are looking for feedback prior to submitting for a grade or the next phase of your project, plan accordingly to give the reader an appropriate time frame to review the material—usually about 1 to 2 weeks.
- **Follow-up.** If you send an email, generally, a response within 48 to 72 hours is customary. Plan ahead with your faculty and understand the process for communicating emergencies. Lack of planning does not constitute an emergency.

LEARNING OBJECTIVES

- Review *The Essentials* (2021) for elements related to professionalism and communication.
- List the areas in which you need to improve.
- Determine the process for communication at your school.

ACTIVITIES

Review the AACN Essentials (2021), with emphasis on Domain 9 and Domain 10. Complete these questions.

1. After reviewing the document, what did you learn?

2. What do you still have questions about?

3. List three sub-competencies in which you feel you need improvement.
   1.
   2.
   3.

In reviewing your syllabus and DNP Program documents, are there any specific processes for communication?

SUMMARY

Knowledge of the Essentials (2021) will help you better engage in conversations with your DNP faculty and DNP team. Clarify any remaining questions with your faculty.

NEXT STEPS

- Discuss your findings with your DNP faculty.

REFERENCES AND RESOURCES

American Association of Colleges of Nursing. (2021). *The essentials: Core competencies for professional nursing education*. https://www.aacnnursing.org/Education-Resources/AACN-Essentials

LESSON 1.2

WRITING A PROFESSIONAL BIO AND GETTING PROFESSIONAL PICTURES

BACKGROUND

If you had to present your entire professional career in one paragraph, what would it say? That is the emphasis of this lesson. Having a professional bio readily available as a DNP student is important. Consider it to be the first impression of who you are and what you have done and highlight your areas of interest.

Bios are used in several ways. You are required to submit the bio when you present at a conference or when you give a guest lecture. Bios are included on websites and social media, such as LinkedIn. Your school will likely utilize your bio when you present your final DNP Project. The bio will need constant updating, but easier to update than start from scratch. A personal bio allows you to highlight your interests, expertise, and the work you have done in a succinct format.

Next you should have a picture to go along with it. We are not talking about a picture of you relaxing on vacation or having a good time at your favorite sporting event. We are talking about a professional headshot, professional poses, well lit, and high resolution. Remember, this is your time to make a first impression—make yourself look the part both online and in person.

As a final thought, business cards are a great networking tool. As a DNP student, we recommend having a card with your name, personal email, and cell phone number on it. You can get a small bundle printed at very minimal cost. Including a QR code may also be useful and technology friendly. Make sure that people know how to connect with you as you seek clinical sites, develop interprofessional relationships, and lead your DNP Project.

LEARNING OBJECTIVES

- Complete your own professional bio.
- Plan/obtain professional photographs.

ACTIVITIES

In this activity, write a draft of your personal bio. Here are some helpful hints and examples.

Helpful Hints:

- Keep it to an appropriate length. Aim for about 10 sentences. However, recognize this may need to be adjusted based on what the bio is for: Twitter/Instagram bios will be short due to space limitations; website bios can be longer; speaker bios will also be relatively short (about 10 sentences).
- Use the appropriate tense. Write your bio in the third person for a more formal tone.
- Remember that this is a living document. The bio will change as your accomplishments and career evolve. Edit and revise your personal bio often to keep it current.
- Showcase your years in healthcare, current role, education (in chronological order), accomplishments, awards, and future endeavors.

Example 1

BIO	NOTES AND OBSERVATIONS
Dr. Agnew began her healthcare career 20 years ago as a CNA just after high school. She graduated from Chicago State University with her bachelors in nursing and is a recent graduate of Bradley University with a Doctorate of Nursing Practice focusing as a Family Nurse Practitioner.	Introduction, years in healthcare. Degrees listed in chronological order.
She has worked in psychiatric nursing, physical rehab, geriatric medicine, addiction rehab, general surgery, orthopedic surgery, neurosurgery, and trauma services both at the bedside and in leadership positions. She currently works in obesity management at the University of Chicago.	Review of clinical experience. Current role.
She is passionate about educating the African American community on preventive health measures such as healthy food choices, exercise, and self-care. Her goal is to continue to serve the underserved population by increasing access to healthcare by opening her own practice.	Goals, projects, future endeavors.

Example 2

BIO	NOTES AND OBSERVATIONS
Dr. Angela Clark received her BSN in 2003 and her MSN in the Perinatal Clinical Nurse Specialist track in 2009 from the University of Kentucky. She received her DNP with an emphasis in Organizational Leadership from Eastern Kentucky University in 2018. Dr. Clark has over 22 years of experience working in obstetrical care including antepartum, intrapartum, postpartum, and newborn nursery. She also currently practices as a staff nurse in the Maternal–Fetal Medicine group at Baptist Health Lexington.	**Education in chronological order.** **Years in healthcare.** **Review of clinical experience.**
Dr. Clark joined the College of Nursing faculty in August 2022 as an Assistant Professor in the undergraduate program as the Course Coordinator for all Maternity and Reproductive Health courses. Previously she was a Senior Clinical Faculty member in the School of Nursing at Eastern Kentucky University and taught for the ASN, traditional and accelerated BSN, RN-BSN, and DNP programs. Teaching experience also includes research for evidence-based nursing practice, DNP role transition, and health promotion.	**Current role.**
Dr. Clark has won awards for her work, including an Eastern Kentucky University's Quality Enhancement Plan Critical Reading Teaching Award in 2022 and the Outstanding Discipline/Application Research Award at the Eastern Kentucky University College of Health Sciences Scholars Day in 2019.	**Awards.**
Dr. Clark is a member of several nursing organizations including Sigma Theta Tau International Honor Society for Nursing, the Association of Women's Health, Obstetric and Neonatal Nursing, the American Association of Nurses, and the Kentucky Association of Nurses.	**Current professional memberships.**

Example 3

BIO	NOTES AND OBSERVATIONS
Karen (Casey) Schill, DNP, APN-C, FNP-BC, ENP-C, CEN, CFRN, NRP, is an assistant professor in the Division of Advanced Nursing Practice in Rutgers School of Nursing. Dr. Schill received her Bachelor's of Nursing degree from Hartwick College in Oneonta, New York. Her career in nursing has focused on emergency nursing and prehospital medicine. She continued her education and received her Family Nurse Practitioner in Emergency Care from Rutgers School of Nursing as well as her DNP at Rutgers School of Nursing. Dr. Schill has more than 20 years of experience in the prehospital setting ranging from basic life support, paramedicine, and air and ground critical care transport. Dr. Schill continues to practice as an emergency nurse practitioner and as a flight nurse.	**Notice use of third person.** **Current academic role.** **Education and career focus.** **Years in healthcare.** **Current clinical role.**

Begin your bio by writing a draft here. Have a colleague review it. Share it with your faculty for input.

Next, use these helpful hints to prepare for your own photographs.

- **Look the part.** Look like the professional you are presenting yourself to be.
- **Use money wisely.** We know students are on a budget. Look to see whether your current employer or school offers the option of professional photos. If not, consider a local photography studio. Your school may also have a marketing or photography department that can help.
- **Choose your clothes carefully.** Wear something you feel confident in. Avoid patterns, seasonal outfits, or clothes you would wear to a party. Remember, this is a picture intended to reflect you as a professional.
- **Use a plain background.** Avoid having a background that may distract from the goal—YOU.
- **The angle.** Consider a universally flattering angle where your body is turned slightly to the left or right with your head turned toward the camera. Always remember to smile!

SUMMARY

Having a professional bio and photograph readily available will be useful in your doctoral work. Remember to proofread the bio and look at other examples for inspiration.

NEXT STEPS

- Finalize your bio.
- Select your professional photo.

REFERENCES AND RESOURCES

American Association of Colleges of Nursing. (2021). *The essentials: Core competencies for professional nursing education.* https://www.aacnnursing.org/Education-Resources/AACN-Essentials

LESSON 1.3

RÉSUMÉ VERSUS CURRICULUM VITAE

BACKGROUND

The DNP degree gives you advanced opportunities. You need to be prepared to reach out to potential collaborators, colleagues, employers, and organizations. Having a curriculum vitae (CV) that is well written affords you the opportunity to showcase why you are a good fit for the organization.

Résumés are summative and generally shorter, no longer than one to two pages. CVs are longer and provide a more thorough, comprehensive summary of your accomplishments. Think of them more as a collective log of all of your professional accomplishments. There is no page limit on a CV. However, it should be organized in a logical manner.

Getting the DNP degree will give you content for your CV. For example, if you are giving a presentation on value-based care in class, consider doing that presentation at a local event. If you are creating an academic poster for class, could it be submitted to a conference? Write a blog for your school or a professional journal. Much of your coursework could be revitalized for dissemination. Talk about this more with your faculty.

LEARNING OBJECTIVES

- Use your résumé to start/revise your CV.
- Plan opportunities to create content for your CV.

ACTIVITIES

In this activity, we want you to start and/or update your CV. Here are some helpful hints:

Helpful Hints

- **Keep it simple.** Avoid a cute, creative font. Choose one that is simple and easy to read. Consider using Times New Roman, Arial, Calibri, or Cambria, for example.
- **Use an appropriate font size.** Keep the text at 11 or 12 points. Your name and section headers can be slightly larger at 14 or 16 points.
- **Consistency is critical.** If you are underlining section titles, do so for all of them.
- **Formatting is important.** White space is a good thing. Keep margins consistent (1 inch on all sides is standard).
- **Organize in sections.** Include contact information (including email, website, phone number, etc.); education; work experience; presentations/publications; research experience; licensure/certifications; awards; and additional training/skills, including additional languages spoken.
- **Review examples for inspiration.** Templates are a great way to get started. Be sure to review examples to give you ideas.

10 The DNP Project Workbook

Exemplar

We present this exemplar for your review. These are the things we feel are well executed in this DNP Student CV:

- Excellent professional photograph
- Clear contact information
- Purposeful opening remark
- Good use of space
- Well organized
- What additional elements appeal to you?

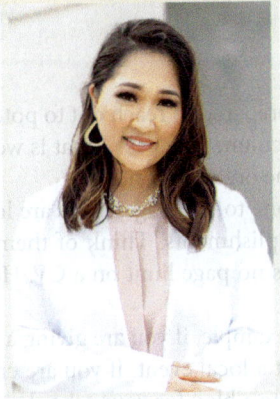

Vanessa A. Abacan, DNP, APRN, ACCNS-P, RNC-MNN, EBP-C

Doctoral-prepared experienced Registered Nurse with a demonstrated expertise in Maternal-Newborn Care, Quality Improvement, Patient Safety, Interdisciplinary Collaboration, and Evidence-Based Practice with a passion in improving patient outcomes. Clinical Nurse Specialist practicum experience include pediatric CVICU, NICU, PICU, and Emergency. Strong experience in Root Cause Analysis and debriefing that fosters psychological safety.

EDUCATION

DOCTOR OF NURSING PRACTICE - CLINICAL NURSE SPECIALIST PEDIATRIC CRITICAL CARE
JOHNS HOPKINS UNIVERSITY SCHOOL OF NURSING
Fall 2018 - Spring 2023
- GPA: 3.77
- Recipient of The Johns Hopkins Nurses' Alumni Association Award
- Doctor of Nursing Practice Conway Scholar
- Sigma Theta Tau Honor Society of Nursing Member
- Nurse Faculty Loan Program Grant Recipient
- Dean's Fund Recipient - 2023

BACHELOR OF SCIENCE IN NURSING
UNIVERSITY OF TEXAS AT ARLINGTON
Spring 2013 - Fall 2016
- Summa Cum Laude

WORK EXPERIENCE

PATIENT SAFETY SPECIALIST
Texas Children's Hospital | November 2021 - present
- Patient Safety Specialist for the Pavilion for Women with 16 floors, 102 patient beds serving patients with high-risk pregnancies in the region.
- Oversee the following units: Labor & Delivery, CCU, Women's Specialty Unit, Women's Assessment Center/Triage, 2 Mother-Baby Units, Perioperative Services, Newborn Nursery, and Milk Bank
- Lead service-wide Pavilion for Women Daily Safety Brief
- Perform monthly Early Elective Delivery audits
- Perform monthly Maternal Early Warning Signs (MEWS) audits on provider responsiveness
- Review safety events submitted through reporting system RL Datix scored per HPI classification, sentinel event criteria, and state reportable events
- Assess for risk, safety threats, level of harm, system opportunities, and identification of trends.
- Lead Root Cause Analyses (RCA) in partnership with Risk Management for all serious safety events and sentinel events. Conduct staff interviews for RCAs
- Create RCA Action Plans within 45 days from commission
- Lead formal staff debriefs for difficult and complicated events to facilitate systems learning
- Present at department-based and hospital-wide meetings on debrief, RCAs system learning
- Advanced Quality Improvement Program - worked with a team of a physician, Clinical Specialist, and support on an NTSV Checklist to reduce NTSV rates at TCH
- Presented on Quality and Safety Principles at a Leadership and New Hire HAC Didactic Education
- Participated as part of the Steering Team for Executive Culture Rounds project
- Participate as one of the Team Leads collaborating with the Chief Quality Officer on Breastfeeding Equity Project

CONTACT
- (281) 709-8309
- drvabacan@gmail.com
- https://portfolium.com/valinsu1
- https://www.linkedin.com/in/vanessa-abacan/

SKILLS
Bilingual (Filipino, English)
Microsoft Office (Word, Excel, PowerPoint, Outlook, Teams, SharePoint)
Project Management
Quality Improvement
Evidence-Based Practice

ORGANIZATIONS
Sigma Theta Tau Honor Society of Nursing – Nu Beta at-Large Chapter
Texas Clinical Nurse Specialists
American Association of Critical-Care Nurses
Association of Women's Health, Obstetric and Neonatal Nurses
National Association of Clinical Nurse Specialists

CERTIFICATIONS
Maternal-Newborn Nursing (RNC-MNN)
Evidence-Based Practice (EBP-C)
BLS
PALS
Advanced Quality Improvement (AQI - certified through TCH)

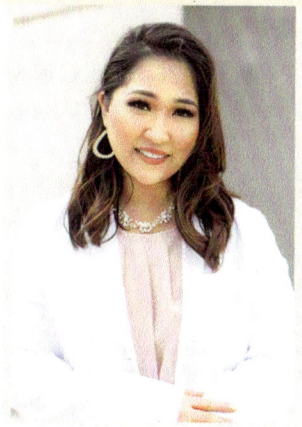

Vanessa A. Abacan, DNP, APRN, ACCNS-P, RNC-MNN, EBP-C

CONTACT

- 📞 (281) 709-8309
- ✉️ drvabacan@gmail.com
- 🌐 https://portfolium.com/valinsu1
- 🌐 https://www.linkedin.com/in/vanessa-abacan/

COMMITTEES

Texas Children's Hospital
- Evidence-Based Practice and Research Council
- Executive Culture Rounds Steering Team
- DNP Collaborative
- Quality Assessment and Performance Improvement
- Publication Task Force
- Breastmilk Feeding Taskforce
- Texas AIM Work Group
- PFW Quality Improvement Work Group
- Skin-to-Skin Task Force

WORK EXPERIENCE

TEACHING ASSISTANT
Johns Hopkins University School of Nursing | January 2023 - present
- Translating Evidence in Practice
- Faculty team of 5 professors
- Grading group of 10 students for all course assignments
- Created a shared Excel Spreadsheet accessible to all course faculty to track students and approved extensions

RN II – MOTHER-BABY UNIT
Houston Methodist West| June 2015 - October 2021
- Assess increasingly complex postpartum patients including postpartum hemorrhage, magnesium sulfate titration/infusion for preeclampsia, HELLP prevention, seizure precautions, drug-positive mothers, postpartum depression prevention/early detection, and fetal demise
- Provide care to newborn babies post transition period including hypoglycemia protocol, educating parents on basic infant care, hypothermia prevention, feeding on demand, baby-friendly implications, jaundice, Coombs positive, ABO incompatibility, period of purple crying, shaken baby syndrome, fall safety precautions
- Collaborate with interdisciplinary team to develop plan of care for patient; making appropriate referrals such as social work, CPS, chaplain etc. as necessary
- Establish partnership with patient - education on postpartum care and infant care
- Support breastfeeding mothers - latching, positioning, and providing breastfeeding aids as appropriate with instruction such as breast pumps, nipple shields shells, and alternate feedings; educating mothers regarding formula and medical indications for supplementation
- Served as a Breastfeeding Unit Champion
- Cross-trained to float to NICU level II – care for feeder growers, withdrawal babies (Neonatal Abstinence Syndrome scoring), IV therapy, venipuncture blood draw, IV catheterization
  - **April 2020 - May 2020 – Labor Pool RN**
    - Assisted as float RN in Emergency Department and HIDU during COVID peak; care across lifespan in ED in collaboration with interdisciplinary team in isolation and COVID management

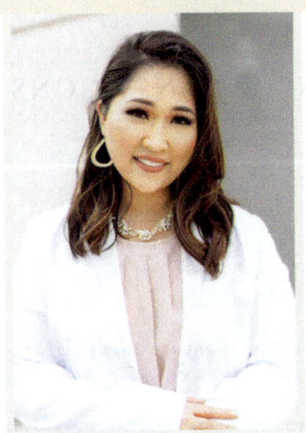

Vanessa A. Abacan, DNP, APRN, ACCNS-P, RNC-MNN, EBP-C

CONTACT

- (281) 709-8309
- drvabacan@gmail.com
- https://portfolium.com/valinsu1
- https://www.linkedin.com/in/vanessa-abacan/

WORK EXPERIENCE

RN II – FAMILY LIFE CENTER (MOTHER-BABY)

Memorial Hermann Healthcare System (Memorial City)| 2014 - 2015

- Assess increasingly complex postpartum patients including postpartum hemorrhage, magnesium sulfate titration/infusion for preeclampsia, HELLP prevention, seizure precautions, drug-positive mothers, postpartum depression prevention/early detection, and fetal demise
- Provide care to newborn babies post transition period including hypoglycemia protocol, educating parents on basic infant care, hypothermia prevention, feeding on demand, baby-friendly implications, jaundice, Coombs positive, ABO incompatibility, period of purple crying, shaken baby syndrome, fall safety precautions
- Collaborate with interdisciplinary team to develop plan of care for patient; making appropriate referrals such as social work, CPS, chaplain etc. as necessary
- Establish partnership with patient - education on postpartum care and infant care
- Support breastfeeding mothers - latching, positioning, and providing breastfeeding aids as appropriate with instruction such as breast pumps, nipple shields shells, and alternate feedings; educating mothers regarding formula and medical indications for supplementation
- Hand Hygiene Unit Auditor
- Blood Transfusion Bridge Medical Super User

GRADUATE NURSE RESIDENCY

North Cypress Medical Center / June 2013 - February 2014

- Provide holistic nursing care to adult/geriatric patients
- Develop plan of care in partnership with the patient as well as family members
- Application of nursing process to develop individualized patient care plan based on needs and priorities
- Address core measures and ensure compliance throughout patient hospital stay
- Evaluate effectiveness of interventions, advocate for patient, and make appropriate referrals
- Recognize changes in patient condition to facilitate prompt and appropriate response
- Educate patients and support person(s) on discharge instructions, medication side effects, compliance, dietary recommendations, signs and symptoms of exacerbation or complication, etc.

Vanessa A. Abacan, DNP, APRN, ACCNS-P, RNC-MNN, EBP-C

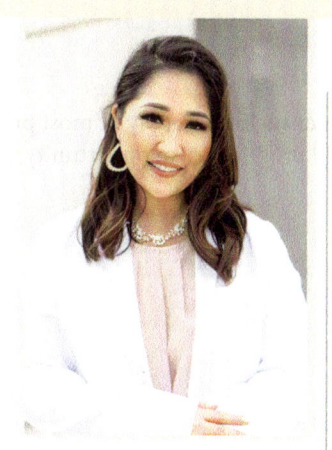

CONTACT

- (281) 709-8309
- drvabacan@gmail.com
- https://portfolium.com/valinsu1
- https://www.linkedin.com/in/vanessa-abacan/

CURRENT PROJECTS

FIRST AUTHOR - Systematic Integrative Review Manuscript "Postpartum sleep and Ramifications on the Maternal-Infant Dyad"
Co-author: Jennie Peterson, PhD, APRN-CNS, CCNS, FAHA

FIRST AUTHOR - Quality Improvement Manuscript "First Touch" - Improving Intraoperative Skin-to-Skin
Co-author: Deborah W. Busch, DNP, CPNP-PC, IBCLC, CNE, FAANP, FAAN

Breastfeeding Equity

Skin-to-Skin Documentation

ACHIEVEMENTS AND RECOGNITIONS

The Johns Hopkins Nurses' Alumni Association Award
DNP Advanced Practice student demonstrating expertise in professional nursing practice and patient-centered health care delivery
May 2023

Accepted as Poster Presentation - Preserving the "First Touch" Intraoperative Skin-to-Skin
Texas Clinical Nurse Specialists Conference
Roundrock, TX / *June 2023*

Accepted as Podium Speaker - "First Touch" Intraoperative Skin-to-Skin
Professional Day Summit
Jan and Dan Duncan Neurological Research Institute (Broadcasted to TCH Woodlands and TCH West Campuses) / *August 2023*

Dean's Travel Fund Recipient
Featured in the Johns Hopkins Nursing Magazine homepage
Johns Hopkins SON / *April 2023*

Patient Safety Liaison/ Team Lead
Patient Safety Week 2023 - "Falling Into Safety"
Team (NICU II) won the Patient Safety Week Poster Contest

One of the Poster Authors - Executive Culture Rounds
Accepted at the IHI Patient Safety Congress 2023

Poster Presenter - "First Touch" Intraoperative Skin-to-Skin
National Association of Clinical Nurse Specialists (NACNS) Conference - Advocacy 2023
Portland, OR / *March 2023*

DAISY Team Awardee
Houston Methodist West / 2019

Featured on the Centennial Wall – "Meaning of Nursing"
Houston Methodist West / 2019

Featured in the Houston Methodist Magazine Winter 2016 Cover Story – "Working with Families"
Houston Methodist West / 2016

Narrative on "Professional Development and Preceptors" for MAGNET Clinical Pathway of Excellence
Houston Methodist West / 2017

Designed pilot for Unit Improvement and Innovation approved for hospital-wide implementation – "Medication Side Effects patient education"
Houston Methodist West / 2018

SUMMARY

At the doctoral level, you will be expected to present a CV. Résumés no longer apply in most professional circumstances. Use these hints to develop your CV. Use your DNP program as an opportunity to develop content for dissemination.

NEXT STEPS

- Develop your CV.
- Create opportunities for dissemination of your DNP work.

REFERENCES AND RESOURCES

American Association of Colleges of Nursing. (2021). *The essentials: Core competencies for professional nursing education.* https://www.aacnnursing.org/Education-Resources/AACN-Essentials

LESSON 1.4

ASSESSMENT OF PERSONAL LEARNING AND LEADERSHIP STYLE

BACKGROUND

Understanding your learning style facilitates success. Although many assessments are available to determine one's learning style, we recommend starting with the VARK Learning Inventory. The inventory is a simple, free online test that gives you results on the way you learn best.

Also consider your leadership style. Just as learning style varies, so does leadership style. No way is the "right" way, but certainly some methods are more effective than others depending on the circumstances. It is important to recognize the different types of leadership and how these impact those being led. We outline next different types of leadership styles and historical figures past and present who have been identified with a specific leadership style.

- **Authoritarian:** Needs individual control of all decisions. "What I say goes." Minimal to no input from others. For example, Bill Gates (Microsoft), Martha Stewart (American businesswoman).
- **Laissez-Faire:** A hands-off approach to leadership in which others are the decision-makers. Can surround themselves with experts who can get the job done. Conversely, sometimes this leadership style can have the opposite result and productivity is very low. For example, Andrew Mellon (industrialist/philanthropist), Ronald Reagan (U.S. president), Steve Jobs (Apple).

- **Democratic**: Leader works together with others during the decision-making process. For example, George Washington (U.S. president), Nelson Mandela (activist and politician).
- **Bureaucratic**: Leadership follows a strict hierarchy with clear rules and positions of power. For example, Winston Churchill (British prime minister), Colin Powell (former U.S. secretary of state).
- **Charismatic**: Relies on charm and charisma to influence people using the art of persuasion. These leaders use their conviction and commitment as their motivation. For example, Mother Teresa (missionary), Lee Iacocca (Chrysler Motors), Barack Obama (former U.S. president).
- **Transformational**: Leader and teamwork together toward a common goal and "big picture." For example, Martin Luther King, Jr. (American minister), Walt Disney (Disney).
- **Servant Leadership**: The leader is successful by serving others in promotion of well-being.

LEARNING OBJECTIVES

- Complete the VARK Inventory.
- Complete a leadership assessment of your choosing.
- Reflect on your results.

ACTIVITIES

Complete your VARK Learning Inventory at https://vark-learn.com/the-vark-questionnaire/.

My Results:

Complete a leadership assessment of your choosing.

My Results:

HINT: The American Organization for Nursing Leadership (AONL) has resources for assessing your ability as a nurse leader. They also have leadership competencies available to review. Most DNP students, regardless of their leadership role, can likely relate to the competencies outlined for population health. The information can be further explored at: https://www.aonl.org/resources/nurse-leader-competencies.

SUMMARY

Stay encouraged as you learn, lead, and complete this DNP Project.

- **Be inspired.** Think about what is important to you and what inspires you. Use this as motivation and create goals. Use that motivation to lead your team.
- **Appeal to your team.** Your goals must align with the goals of those you hope will follow.
- **Reward and recognize achievement.** Whether the victories are small or big, celebrate and reward accomplishments. The positive reinforcement will keep you motivated.
- **Keep going.** Don't give up. Setbacks will happen, but a true leader will persevere.

NEXT STEPS

- Use your VARK results in your learning process.
- Continue to develop your leadership skills.

REFERENCES AND RESOURCES

American Association of Colleges of Nursing. (2021). *The essentials: Core competencies for professional nursing education.* https://www.aacnnursing.org/Education-Resources/AACN-Essentials

American Organization for Nursing Leadership. (2023). *AONL nurse leader core competencies.* https://www.aonl.org/resources/nurse-leader-competencies

LESSON 1.5

DEVELOPING BASIC TECHNOLOGY SKILLS FOR THE DNP PROJECT

BACKGROUND

Basic technology skills are a requirement for the DNP Project. The skills identified here are not generally skills that are taught as part of the program. Rather they are skills you learn/refine on your own. It is very common for DNP students to start their program and then feel overwhelmed when they are asked to complete assignments that require technology. It behooves you to become familiar with these computer programs as early in your DNP program as possible. Although it will take some time on the front end to learn, this investment will pay off 10-fold on the back end when the programs can work for you and make life much easier. Talk to your DNP faculty about preferences for technology. Some software may be offered free of charge through your school. Resources may also be available through the libraries that teach you how to use key software programs.

LEARNING OBJECTIVES

- List potential technology skills.
- Develop a plan to become competent.

ACTIVITIES

Following are some suggested activities. Review the list and then identify three skills to master prior to starting your DNP Project.

Suggestions:

- Familiarize yourself with word-processing programs: Microsoft Word, Google Docs, and so on.
- Key skills:
  - Creating a table of contents using levels of headings
  - Formatting/inserting tables and figures
  - Creating hanging indents for reference pages (for those required to use American Psychological Association [APA])
  - Proper use of page and section breaks
  - Integrating EndNote/RefWorks/Zotero into your documents
  - Familiarize yourself with data-management systems: Microsoft Excel, Google Sheets, SPSS, and so on
- Key skills:
  - Data entry
  - Creating graphs and tables from data sets
  - Use of basic formulas for data analysis
  - Familiarize yourself with presentation software: Microsoft PowerPoint, Google Slides, Prezi, and so on
- Key skills:
  - Professional presentation design; proper use of images, art
  - Use of notes section
  - Use of presenter mode (for schools with projection abilities)
  - How to embed videos
  - Familiarize yourself with citation management software: EndNote, RefWorks, Zotero, and so on
- Key skills:
  - How to import/export citations
  - Use of EndNote/RefWorks in Word to "cite as you write"
  - How to change formatting for different reference styles

Based on this review, I need to improve on:

1.

2.

3.

SUMMARY

Mastering technology skills early in the DNP Project process will set you up for success.

NEXT STEPS

- Develop a plan to address your identified gaps.

REFERENCES AND RESOURCES

American Association of Colleges of Nursing. (2021). *The essentials: Core competencies for professional nursing education.* https://www.aacnnursing.org/Education-Resources/AACN-Essentials

LESSON 1.6

DEVELOPING WRITING SKILLS

BACKGROUND

The DNP Project and other doctoral work require high-level scholarly writing. If you struggle with academic writing, seek help early and often. Many schools provide resources for graduate students. Reading examples of scholarly works also informs one's writing. However, we observe that students fail to take advantage of these services, or seek outside services, in a timely manner. Writing requires practice and time. It is imperative to establish good writing habits as a doctoral student.

LEARNING OBJECTIVES

- Consider suggestions for establishing good writing habits.
- Determine resources for writing support.

ACTIVITIES

What is your writing process? The following suggestions are from DNP faculty. After you review them, list three actions you will take to establish good writing habits.

DNP faculty suggestions:

- **Workspace**: Establish a designated workspace where you will go when you are ready to write.
- **Make it a date**: Set writing goals on your calendar. Block time for writing.
- **Draft an outline first**: Look at the rubric of your assignment. Make an outline that addresses each point before you write.

- **Stay on schedule**: In your writing block, use a timer to stay focused. When the timer goes off, get up and move. As scheduled, go back for another round.
- **Block social media and notifications**. Multiple distractions will impede your progress. Turn notifications off when you write.
- **Keep track:** Track your writing time when you are done.
- **Use the buddy system:** Get an accountability partner for writing. Check in or text them when you've finished writing and tell them how long you worked.
- **Proofread**: Despite feeling like you know your paper inside and out, proofread it. In fact, have someone else read it. The challenge is that we know what it is supposed to say, but that doesn't mean that is what it actually says.
- **Know your limitations**: Although it is a large investment, consider the possibility of using your college's/university's writing center or even hiring an editor. For example, editing jobs can be posted online using sites like *UpWork*. You describe what you need done and what you will pay. People can bid on the job. Ask your faculty about editing services they recommend.
- **Back up your files**: Save your documents to a flash drive or a cloud account, email them to yourself, and so on. Consider the situation of a friend whose car was broken into. Not only was their laptop (with the project paper on it) stolen but so was the flash drive containing the only other versions of the project.
- **Name your files appropriately**: Include your last name, date, and keyword/phrase in the file name. If you just save files by course or week of the assignment, you may not be able to find things later.
- **Expect multiple drafts and revisions:** Recognizing scholarly writing is an iterative process is imperative. The first draft is just that—a first draft. You'll likely have several versions of your paper over the course of writing it. When you think it is as good as it can be, you'll receive feedback for improving it even further.

SUMMARY

Develop good writing habits in your DNP program. Use resources available to you for success.

NEXT STEPS

- Establish your writing habits.
- Use available resources.

REFERENCES AND RESOURCES

American Association of Colleges of Nursing. (2021). *The essentials: Core competencies for professional nursing education.* https://www.aacnnursing.org/Education-Resources/AACN-Essentials

LESSON 1.7

TIME MANAGEMENT STRATEGIES

BACKGROUND

In most cases, DNP students are often juggling a variety of responsibilities while attending school and completing their DNP Project. Careers, children, spouses, partners, friends, and even parents or grandchildren are all vying for your attention. It's hard to say no, but recognizing the need to find balance is important. The DNP program and DNP Project will take your time and energy. Plan for it.

LEARNING OBJECTIVES

- Develop a detailed schedule.

ACTIVITIES

Review these helpful hints regarding time management. Highlight things that stand out to you. Then, complete a short reflection.

Time management strategies:

- **Be committed:** Once you sit down to work, commit to staying with it for the time you set aside. Avoid distractions during this time—do not check emails, take phone calls, or check social media. If this is time set aside for schoolwork, then keep it that way.
- **Keep a schedule**: Planning out a timeline and sticking to it help create some accountability. Be very detailed as you plan. Include work, home, and school. Make time for self-care as well.
- **Schedule time to think**: You will not be innovative if you are exhausted.
- **Prioritize your work.** The work that rises to the top of the to-do list should be done first.
- **Say no**. Recognize that "No." is a complete sentence. You do not need a reason to say no. Sometimes saying no is the best way to ensure your work gets completed. Avoid overcommitment. Saying yes to something is time taken away from writing your DNP Project proposal/final project.
- **Plan ahead:** Plan your weeks ahead of time. Start on Sunday and figure out what needs to be accomplished. This allows you to focus and set goals for the week's activities.
- **Schedule breaks:** Planning for a break periodically helps you avoid burnout.
- **Take care of yourself.** This means both physically and mentally. Physical activity like exercise or yoga is helpful. Also important is to make sure you get enough sleep. This also includes setting aside some relaxation time.
- **Delegate**: If there are tasks that can be delegated, do so!

Reflection:

- What items from this list stand out or apply to your circumstances?
- What actions will you take to utilize your time wisely while completing your DNP Project?

NEXT STEPS

- Develop a schedule for efficient use of time.

REFERENCES AND RESOURCES

American Association of Colleges of Nursing. (2021). *The essentials: Core competencies for professional nursing education.* https://www.aacnnursing.org/Education-Resources/AACN-Essentials

CHAPTER SUMMARY

You are now set up for success! Remember to continue to develop these skills as you work toward your terminal degree. The DNP journey is more than just the project. It is a pathway for self-development, a change of career trajectory, and a new level of professionalism. As a result of engaging in this work, you can

- Communicate at the appropriate level in a professional manner.
- Present a professional identity in various formats.
- Continue to demonstrate competency in writing, time management, and use of emotional intelligence.

Let's get started on the next chapter!

2

Understanding the DNP Degree and DNP Project

Editors: Brenda Douglass and Sharon Stager
Contributors: Molly Bradshaw, Tracy R. Vitale, Rachel Risner, Sallie Porter, Melissa deCardi Hladek, Deborah Busch, Lisa Grubb, Kimberly McIltrot, Jessica Dean Murphy, Ashly Ninan, Susan Renda, Martha Abshire Saylor, and Brigit VanGraafeiland

Lessons

Lesson 2.1	Why Get a Terminal Degree?
Lesson 2.2	Nursing Degree Versus Nursing Role
Lesson 2.3	Understanding the Essentials
Lesson 2.4	Comparing the DNP and PhD
Lesson 2.5	Evidence-Based Practice and Quality Improvement
Lesson 2.6	What Is a DNP Project?
Lesson 2.7	Design Types of DNP Projects
Lesson 2.8	DNP Project Requirements at Your School
Lesson 2.9	Review of Completed DNP Projects
Lesson 2.10	The DNP Experience and Practice Hours
Lesson 2.11	Group DNP Projects

OBJECTIVES

The purpose of this chapter is to introduce fundamental concepts of the DNP degree and the DNP Project. The student will complete a series of lessons designed to introduce basic information that is necessary to start the process of the DNP Project.

By the end of this chapter, you will be able to

- Compare and contrast the DNP and PhD terminal degrees in the context of nursing roles.
- Analyze the minimum requirements of a DNP Project.
- Critique DNP Projects to examine content.

INTRODUCTION

The DNP Project process begins with establishing a solid foundation. In this chapter, fundamental documents are introduced that inform the requirements of the DNP degree and DNP Project. These documents are vital to understand and complete the activities presented in the sequential lessons as the activities build upon one another. Each lesson is broken down into manageable segments.

In this process, the chapter activities will present key concepts that you will need to understand for the DNP degree and project. While some activities may be perceived as repetitive, the lessons will inform you of the requirements necessary to fulfill the DNP degree.

These lessons call for you to include and partner with your faculty. To streamline your efforts, a foundation to fine-tune and focus on the principles of the DNP Project are provided in this chapter. There are specific competencies to achieve when completing an advanced degree. There are 10 domains within the *Essentials* (American Association of Colleges of Nursing [AACN], 2021). These competencies will be threaded through a DNP curriculum, and you will be expected to demonstrate mastery with the DNP Project. A DNP graduate is expected to master the Advanced-Level competencies and sub-competencies delineated within the *Essentials* (AACN, 2021). You will become familiar with this content as we work.

The DNP is a terminal practice degree in nursing. Recognizing the degree preparation for DNP and PhD is important to articulate and differentiate. While the DNP is practice-focused, the PhD is research-focused (AACN, 2006). Historically, the PhD and Nursing Doctorate (ND) degrees were the only terminal degree in nursing. The EdD in nursing education has been available. Some DNP programs are also offering a DNP with an emphasis on education. Be clear of the focus of your program prior to starting. In a DNP program, you will *not* be generating new research; rather, you will be conducting a systematic scientific method process to evaluate evidence and translate it into practice.

The DNP Project at its core is a supervised, high-level problem-solving process. The DNP student must identify problems, assess the situation, and use evidence to develop, implement, and evaluate outcomes and process. Our solutions must be sustainable and designed to impact the patients we serve. The inquiry is not a one and done experience. The first experience in conducting a scientific methods project may require mentoring. The expectation is for the experience to inspire you to continue questioning practice, while engaging in change and enhancing health outcomes. The process is rooted in evidence-based practice and quality improvement.

The DNP Project is about taking research that already exists, evaluating it, and finding ways to translate, implement, and utilize it within the practice setting. Did you know that it takes 17 years to translate research into practice (Morris et al., 2011)? Our PhD prepared colleagues take the lead of generating nursing research. They are the experts of nursing science. We, the DNPs, with PhDs take the lead by deciding how to translate, utilize, and evaluate the impact of that research on patients because we are the experts of nursing practice (AACN, 2015).

At the conclusion of the chapter, we dive into the development of a DNP Project. We guide you through the expectations for DNP Projects, as outlined by the AACN and help you prepare questions for faculty as you review the project expectations at your school. Most importantly, we review some projects together. The chapter ends with some suggestions and clarification on group DNP Projects.

Start here and work hard, so that you can finish strong. Let's begin.

REFERENCES AND RESOURCES

American Association of Colleges of Nursing. (2006). *The essentials of doctoral education for advanced nursing practice.* https://www.aacnnursing.org/Portals/42/Publications/DNPEssentials.pdf

American Association of Colleges of Nursing. (2015). *The doctor of nursing practice: Current issues and clarifying recommendations. [White paper].* https://www.aacnnursing.org/Portals/42/News/White-Papers/DNP-Implementation-TF-Report-8-15.pdf

American Association of Colleges of Nursing. (2021). *The essentials: Core competencies for professional nursing education.* https://www.aacnnursing.org/Education-Resources/AACN-Essentials

Morris, Z. S., Wooding, S., & Grant, J. (2011). The answer is 17 years, what is the question: Understanding time lags in translational research. *Journal of the Royal Society of Medicine, 104*(12), 510–520.

MY GOALS FOR UNDERSTANDING THE DNP DEGREE AND DNP PROJECT ARE TO:

_____
_____
_____
_____
_____
_____
_____
_____
_____
_____
_____
_____
_____
_____
_____
_____
_____
_____
_____
_____
_____
_____
_____

LESSON 2.1

WHY GET A TERMINAL DEGREE?

BACKGROUND

The Institute of Medicine's (IOM, 2011a) report *The Future of Nursing* offers a true vision for the evolution of nursing practice. This report specifically calls for nurses to be prepared at the highest level of nursing practice beyond the initial preparation in the discipline (IOM, 2011a). The DNP is a terminal nursing *practice* degree designed to equip nurses for the highest levels of practice and leadership, to drive change and improve health outcomes (American Association of Colleges of Nursing [AACN], 2004). To gain perspective around *The Future of Nursing* report (IOM, 2011a), it is imperative to understand many facets surrounding the DNP degree. At this point, it is important to understand the DNP degree and why this degree is necessary to your professional growth and development. Why are you pursuing the DNP degree? Nursing skill sets evolve over time. What skills will the DNP add to your nursing practice? Nurses need advanced-level knowledge and skill sets to navigate and solve problems in complex healthcare environments. The DNP-prepared nurse is required to have a broad perspective to evaluate and navigate the healthcare climate of today. Nurses need to lead and *practice* at the highest level.

LEARNING OBJECTIVES

- Distinguish the DNP degree from other terminal nursing degrees.
- Articulate why the DNP degree is necessary for nursing's future and your future.
- Utilize AACN's *The Essentials* (2021) to identify key goals for knowledge and skill sets in pursuing a DNP degree.

ACTIVITIES

Read the IOM (2011b), *Future of Nursing* report brief, the AACN's (2004) position statement on DNP education, and the AACN *Essentials* (2021). List the key points regarding DNP education. Seek additional perspectives by engaging in discussions with nursing leaders, educators, and peers.

The Future of Nursing report brief describes four key messages. Identify the four key messages in the spaces provided.

1.

2.

3.

4.

☑ Other Notes: *The Future of Nursing* Report

The AACN (2004) Position Statement on the Practice Doctorate in Nursing describes the climate of nursing at the time. The position statement provides a greater understanding of the evolution regarding the DNP degree. After exploring the position statement, define the three major categories of "practice" in the spaces provided.

1.

2.

3.

☑ Incorporate the current perspectives of the Practice Doctorate in Nursing. Compare and contrast between the "practice-focused" DNP degree and the "research-focused" PhD degree? Complete the chart. The first comparison has been completed for you.

DNP: "PRACTICE-FOCUSED" DEGREE	PHD: "RESEARCH-FOCUSED" DEGREE
Less emphasis on theory and metatheory	PhD places more focus on nursing theories

☑ The AACN published revised *Essentials* (2021) to specify competency-based expectations for students, educators, and employers to prepare nursing's future workforce. Review AACN *The Essentials* document (2021), specifically Advanced-Level Nursing Education, to conceptualize the role of the DNP-prepared nurse. Identify five competencies in which the *Essentials* (2021) can facilitate and develop the attributes of a DNP-prepared nurse and inform the DNP Project.

1.

2.

3.

4.

5.

☑ **After examining the IOM (2011b) *Future of Nursing* report brief, the AACN's (2004) position statement on DNP education, and the AACN *Essentials* (2021), reflect and identify on the key aspects of the DNP degree that will promote advanced-level knowledge and skill sets within your practice.**

1.

2.

3.

SUMMARY

The DNP-prepared nurse is a clinical practice expert equipped with knowledge, skills, and attributes to identify problems, draw on evidence-based research to identify potential solutions, and evaluate the impact on healthcare outcomes. The DNP degree provides the nurse with the skill set to work at the highest level of practice and be competent in the expectations outlined within *The Essentials* and aligned to *The Future of Nursing* report (AACN, 2021; IOM, 2011a).

NEXT STEPS

- Discuss your findings in this chapter with nursing leaders, educators, and peers.
- Visit the "Campaign for Action" website (https://campaignforaction.org/about), which includes goals stemming from *The Future of Nursing* (IOM, 2011a) report.
- Read more about the IOM's Future of Nursing Report on Education.
- Review the AACN *Essentials* (2021).

REFERENCES AND RESOURCES

American Association of Colleges of Nursing. (2004). *AACN position statement on the practice doctorate in nursing.* https://www.aacnnursing.org/Portals/42/News/Position-Statements/DNP.pdf

American Association of Colleges of Nursing. (2021). *The essentials: Core competencies for professional nursing education.* https://www.aacnnursing.org/Education-Resources/AACN-Essentials

Institute of Medicine. (2011a). *The future of nursing: Leading change, advancing health.* National Academies Press. https://www.nap.edu/read/12956/chapter/1

Institute of Medicine. (2011b). *Report brief: The future of nursing: Leading change, advancing health.* http://nationalacademies.org/hmd/%7E/media/Files/Report%20Files/2010/The-Future-of-Nursing/Future%20of%20Nursing%202010%20Report%20Brief.pdf

RELATED TEXTBOOK

Dreher, H., & Glasgow, M. (2023). *DNP role development for doctoral advanced nursing practice* (3rd ed.). Springer Publishing Company.

Section I: Historical and Theoretical Foundations for Role Delineation and Preparation in Doctoral Advanced Nursing Practice—Chapters 1, 2, and 3.

LESSON 2.2

NURSING DEGREE VERSUS NURSING ROLE

BACKGROUND

The DNP degree is an academic accomplishment, not a nursing role. The Institute of Medicine's (IOM, 2011) report, *The Future of Nursing: Leading Change, Advancing Health,* highly promotes that nurses are lifelong learners. Nurses should reflect upon their current role and their aspired career trajectory. Nursing has many roles, some of which include staff nurse, nurse manager, nurse executive, or advanced practice nurse. Many roles will require greater knowledge and skill sets which advancing education can satisfy. Licensure requirements are mandated by individual states and need to be understood.

According to AACN (2021), "*The Essentials: Core Competencies for Professional Nursing Education* provides a framework for preparing individuals as members of the discipline of nursing, reflecting expectations across the trajectory of nursing education and applied experience" (p. 2). Pursuing a DNP degree may or may not change your role in nursing. A DNP degree may provide greater opportunities and support your intended goals within the nursing profession. The DNP as a terminal degree prepares the nurse to practice at the highest level of nursing (AACN, 2006, 2021).

LEARNING OBJECTIVES

- Consider the differences between the entry-level and advanced-level nursing education.
- Describe the Consensus Model for Advanced Practice Nursing.

- Review the Consensus Model and state requirement in the location of practice.
- Explore the options for completion of the DNP degree.

ACTIVITY

Examine the options for nursing roles beyond entry-level nursing. Compare and identify your current role and aspired nursing role. What are the knowledge and skill sets required to achieve your aspired goal?

Hint

For this exercise, you are to focus on a practice role in nursing. A nurse educator is required to be an expert in a specific area of nursing. Thus, the nurse educator role will not be appropriate to identify as a current or future nursing role in this exercise. Consider *only* your nursing practice role. All nurses need additional training to achieve the competencies required of a nurse educator (National League for Nursing, 2012). The focus of the DNP degree is to augment and specialize in an area of practice. The nurse educator role is a separate and distinctive role which will be addressed in subsequent lessons.

My current nursing practice role: _____

My aspired nursing practice role: _____

For nurses who are considering a role in advanced practice nursing, it is necessary to understand the requirements of licensure and the Consensus Model for APRN regulation. The National Council of State Boards of Nursing (NCSBN) published the Consensus Model in 2008 for uniformity of licensure, accreditation, certification, and education of the APRN in every state (2023). The goal of this model is to provide unification, standardization, and regulation of these roles across the country.

Review the information on the Consensus Model (www.ncsbn.org/aprn-consensus.htm).

Step 1: Choose your advanced practice nursing role.

Step 2: If applicable, choose your population of focus and complete the required training.

Step 3: Obtain licensure in your state of practice.

Step 4: Specialize further within your role, population, and training via additional education.

Next, fill out your information:

_____
Advanced Practice Training/Specialization

_____
Licensure

_____
Population of Focus

_____
Your Role

Based on your future aspired nursing role, identify your current nursing degree and trajectory to obtain a DNP. Trace the options for completing the DNP degree (Figure 2.1).

Option 1: Practical Nurse (LPN) → Associate Degree in Nursing (ADN) → Baccalaureate Degree in Nursing (BSN) → Master's Degree in Nursing (MSN) → Doctor of Nursing Practice (DNP)

*One goal of *The Future of Nursing* report is to promote life long learning…

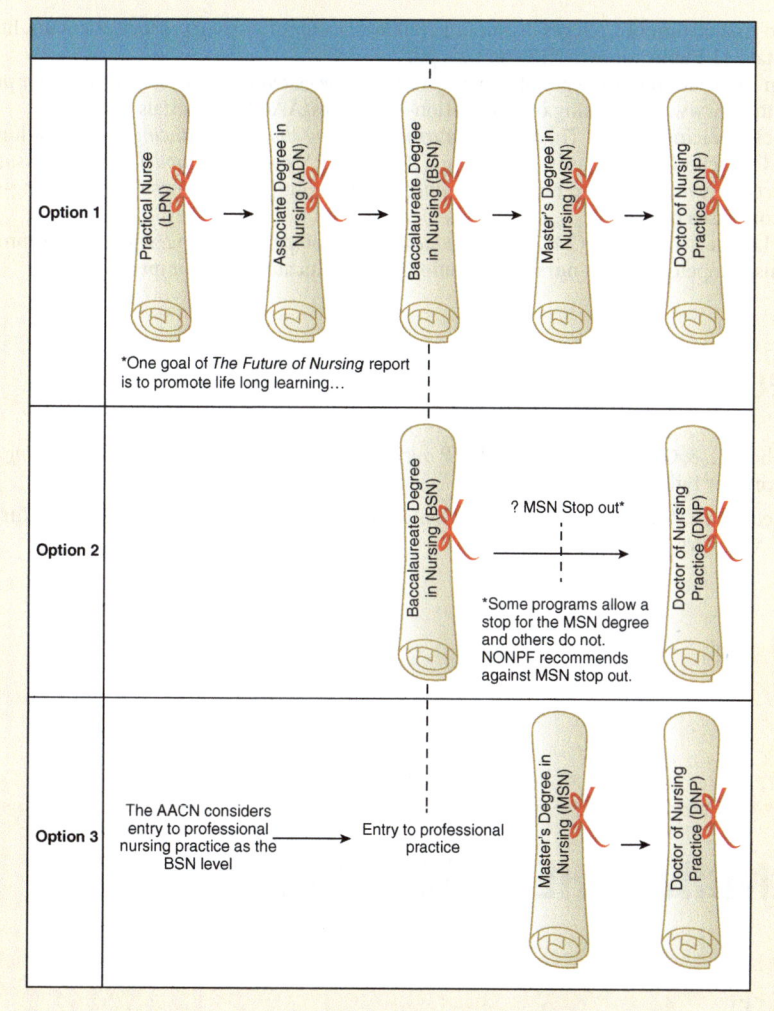

Option 2: Baccalaureate Degree in Nursing (BSN) → ? MSN Stop out* → Doctor of Nursing Practice (DNP)

*Some programs allow a stop for the MSN degree and others do not. NONPF recommends against MSN stop out.

Option 3: The AACN considers entry to professional nursing practice as the BSN level → Entry to professional practice → Master's Degree in Nursing (MSN) → Doctor of Nursing Practice (DNP)

Figure 2.1 Three common pathways to a DNP degree. AACN, American Association of Colleges of Nursing; NONPF, National Organization of Nurse Practitioner Faculties.

SUMMARY

Beyond your current role as a nurse, identify your aspired advanced-level nursing role and the impact of the DNP degree. If this role aligns to an APRN role, ensure that the criterion for licensure is clearly understood for the state in which you plan to practice. In addition, there are national certifying bodies based on population-specific APRN roles. The DNP prepares the professional to practice at the highest level in the nursing discipline.

NEXT STEPS

- Review the Consensus Model and state requirement in the location of practice.
- Discuss this list with nursing leaders, educators, and peers to collaborate and develop an actionable list.

REFERENCES AND RESOURCES

American Association of Colleges of Nursing. (2006). *Doctor of nursing practice essentials.* https://www.aacnnursing.org/Portals/42/Publications/DNPEssentials.pdf

American Association of Colleges of Nursing. (2021). *The essentials: Core competencies for professional nursing education.* https://www.aacnnursing.org/Education-Resources/AACN-Essentials

Institute of Medicine. (2011). *The future of nursing: Leading change, advancing health.* National Academies Press.

National Council of State Boards of Nursing. (2023). *APRN consensus model: The consensus model for APRN regulation, licensure, accreditation, certification and education.* https://www.ncsbn.org/nursing-regulation/practice/aprn/aprn-consensus.page

National League for Nursing. (2012). *Nurse educator core competency.* http://www.nln.org/professional-development-programs/competencies-for-nursing-education/nurse-educator-core-competency

RELATED TEXTBOOK

Dreher, H., & Glasgow, M. (2023). *DNP role development for doctoral advanced nursing practice* (3rd ed.). Springer Publishing Company.

    Section II: Primary and Secondary Contemporary Roles for Doctoral Advanced Nursing Practice—Chapters 6, 7, 8, and 9.

LESSON 2.3

UNDERSTANDING THE ESSENTIALS

BACKGROUND

The American Association of Colleges of Nursing (AACN) is a national organization focused on academic nursing. Collectively, the organization is composed of approximately 865 member schools of nursing, over 52,000 faculty members, and 565,000 students from both public and private universities (AACN, 2023). In collaboration with partnering organizations, the AACN provides a framework of competencies for entry-level and advanced-level nursing practice. The *Essentials* serve to bridge the gap between education and practice, utilizing competency-based education to prepare nurses for the complexity of the healthcare environment of today (AACN, 2021).

The Essentials: Core Competencies for Professional Nursing Education were published in 2021 and are the cornerstone for curriculum (AACN, 2021). These *Essentials* introduce 10 specific domains that represent the key components to be achieved in professional nursing from entry level to advanced level (AACN, 2021). Each domain includes a descriptor (working definition), a contextual statement, and distinguishable competencies at each level of nursing. Within the domains, there are subcompetencies to provide understandable, observable, and measurable criteria (AACN, 2021).

To attain a DNP degree, learners are to demonstrate entry-level and advanced-level competencies and sub-competencies and advanced specialty/role competencies into practice (AACN, 2021). These competencies are not a "one and done" or "checklist approach" (AACN, 2021). The purpose of these competencies is intended for learners to demonstrate attainment of competencies in multiple and authentic contexts over time (AACN, 2021).

In academia, nursing schools are expected to uphold accreditation standards, in which the *Essentials* are a guiding framework in preparing a professional nurse. A scholarly work focused on improving clinical practice is required of students completing a practice doctorate in nursing (AACN, 2021). The process of conducting a DNP Project provides an opportunity for the student to demonstrate new skills into practice and to demonstrate many of the principles of nursing scholarship delineated in the *Essentials* (AACN, 2021). The blending of knowledge, skills, and professional comportment to advanced-level nursing provides opportunity for quality improvement processes, enhancement of healthcare outcomes, systematic and organizational leadership, and translation of evidence-based practice (AACN, 2021).

The project is one way to demonstrate competency of the *Essentials*. The DNP Project is scholarly work, which includes problem identification; an expansive review of literature, analysis, and synthesis; translating evidence to construct a strategy or method to address a problem; designing an implementation plan and actual implementation; and the evaluation of outcomes, processes, and/or experience (AACN, 2021). Execution of the DNP Project requires faculty guidance and supervision (AACN, 2021). Faculty is responsible for evaluation of the final DNP Project (AACN, 2021). The DNP practice experience and practice hours will be discussed in detail in a later activity.

It is imperative to understand the *Essentials*. In this lesson, we introduce the domains of the *Essentials*. The goal is to garner familiarity with the competencies that you will be required to demonstrate and how it impacts the DNP Project. It may be helpful to return to this lesson later as you progress through your DNP program.

LEARNING OBJECTIVES

- Read the AACN's *Essentials* (2021).
- Identify the specific domains and applicable competencies within the AACN *Essentials* (2021) that necessitate greater emphasis to achieve your intended advanced-level goals.
- Develop a list of knowledge and skills based on the AACN *Essentials* Advanced-Level competencies in which you identify areas of opportunities to grow within your new role.
- Identify activities or DNP Project constructs to support scholarly project development and demonstration of competencies aligned to each of the domains within *The Essentials*.
- Prepare questions for faculty to integrate the *Essentials* within your DNP curricular learning activities and the DNP Project.

ACTIVITIES

Read the AACN *Essentials* (2021) document. Examine each of the domains and utilize the following table and descriptors. Determine the activities and the construct for the scholarly DNP Project product to demonstrate the advanced-level competencies. Include a minimum of two activities for each domain. Note a single activity may satisfy more than one competency. Write down any questions you have for your faculty.

Domain 1: Knowledge for Nursing Practice

Activities:

Question(s):

Domain 2: Person-Centered Care

Activities:

Question(s):

34 The DNP Project Workbook

Domain 3: Population Health

Activities:

Question(s):

Domain 4: Scholarship for Nursing Practice

Activities:

Question(s):

Domain 5: Quality and Safety

Activities:

Question(s):

Domain 6: Interprofessional Partnerships

Activities:

Question(s):

Domain 7: Systems-Based Practice

Activities:

Question(s):

Domain 8: Informatics and Healthcare Technologies

Activities:

Question(s):

Domain 9: Professionalism

Activities:

Question(s):

Domain 10: Personal, Professional, and Leadership Development

Activities:

Question(s):

SUMMARY

When reviewing the *Essentials*, evaluate the similarities and differences between the entry-level and advanced-level competencies. The DNP-prepared nurse is empowered, equipped, and prepared for leadership roles. The DNP degree is designed to prepare nurses for the highest levels of practice and leadership, to drive change and improve health outcomes (AACN, 2004).

NEXT STEPS

- Continue work toward mastery of the *Essentials*.
- Consider the *Essentials* as you develop the DNP Project.

REFERENCES AND RESOURCES

American Association of Colleges of Nursing. (2004). *AACN position statement on the practice doctorate in nursing.* https://www.aacnnursing.org/Portals/42/News/Position-Statements/DNP.pdf

American Association of Colleges of Nursing. (2021). *The essentials: Core competencies for professional nursing education.* https://www.aacnnursing.org/Education-Resources/AACN-Essentials

American Association of Colleges of Nursing. (2023). *AACN fact sheets.* https://www.aacnnursing.org/news-data/fact-sheets/aacn-fact-sheet

RELATED TEXTBOOK

Christenbery, T (Ed.). (2018). *Evidence-based practice in nursing.* Springer Publishing Company.
   Preface: Goals of This Book
   Chapter 19: EBP: The Sequential Layering of BSN, MSN, and DNP Competencies and Opportunities
   Table 19.1 AACN EBP Essentials Crosswalk

Dreher, H., & Glasgow, M. (2023). *DNP role development for doctoral advanced nursing practice* (3rd ed.). Springer Publishing Company.
   Section III: Operationalizing Role Functions of Doctoral Advanced Nursing Practice—Chapter 24.

LESSON 2.4

COMPARING THE DNP AND PHD

BACKGROUND

The DNP is an option for a terminal practice degree in nursing. The curriculum for the DNP degree is based on the *Essentials* (American Association of Colleges of Nursing [AACN], 2021). The DNP degree is different than other terminal degree options such as the PhD. The DNP degree does not determine one's nursing role. It ensures that nurses have a skill set to engage in practice at the highest levels of nursing (AACN, 2006, 2021). DNP- and PhD-prepared nurses should collaborate to maximize health-related outcomes.

In this lesson, the DNP degree is compared to other terminal-degree options in nursing, specifically, the PhD. Distinguishing the differences will be key to your own DNP Project. Historically, the DNP Project has been a challenging concept to understand. Students are often unable to articulate the differences. For many students, the "ah-ha" moment may not come until later in their program of study. From the beginning, this lesson plan aims to help clarify the DNP degree compared to the PhD degree.

LEARNING OBJECTIVES

- Outline the components of the DNP degree and PhD degree.
- Compare and contrast the elements of the degrees.

ACTIVITIES

At the most fundamental level, the AACN defines the DNP as a practice-focused degree and the PhD as a research-focused degree. Practice is broadly defined as "any form of nursing intervention that influences healthcare outcomes for individuals or populations" (AACN, 2006, p. 2). The *Essentials* (AACN, 2021) go on to discuss research focus as "knowledge-generating" (AACN, 2006, p. 3) and more intently focused on concepts of theory, methodology, and statistical precision (AACN, 2006). Concepts related to the DNP and PhD degree, respectively, are broken down in the following tables by category. Information from the AACN has been translated into each box for you. Use additional resources to add expand on each concept. Suggested material can be found under "References and Resources" in this section. Be certain to write down questions for discussion with your faculty member.

CONCEPT	DNP (PRACTICE FOCUSED)	PHD (RESEARCH FOCUSED)
Purpose of degree	Prepare nurses at the highest level of nursing *practice*: • Generate knowledge via practice innovation or evidence-based QI[a] • Translate research into practice[b]	Prepare nurses at the highest level of nursing *science*: • Generate new knowledge via application of rigorous scientific methods • Conduct research to advance nursing science
Students	Committed to a career in practice	Committed to a career in research
Program outcomes	Healthcare improvement by: • Practice contributions • Practice scholarship • Policy changes • Leadership in practice	Healthcare improvement by: • Scientific contributions • Scientific scholarship • Scientific inquiry • Leadership in research
Notes:		

[a]QI, quality improvement. Remember that these are nursing degrees, and they are not nursing roles.
[b]All nurses will complete additional training to prepare them for their nursing roles.

Source: Data from the American Association of Colleges of Nursing. (2021). *The essentials: Core competencies for professional nursing education.* https://www.aacnnursing.org/Education-Resources/AACN-Essentials; American Association of Colleges of Nursing. (2015). *The doctor of nursing practice: Current issues and clarifying recommendations* [White paper]. https://www.aacnnursing.org/Portals/42/News/White-Papers/DNP-Implementation-TF-Report-8-15.pdf.

CONCEPT	DNP (PRACTICE FOCUSED)	PHD (RESEARCH FOCUSED)
Final academic product	DNP Project	Dissertation
Faculty/experts advising the student	DNP Team	Committee
Intention	The DNP Project is a learning experience. The DNP Project is meant to improve outcomes in a local context/population: • Transferrable outcomes • One project cycle/degree	The PhD dissertation is a learning experience. The PhD dissertation is meant to provide information that can be generalized to a larger context/population: • Generalizable outcomes • Large study with multiple manuscripts/degree

CONCEPT	DNP (PRACTICE FOCUSED)	PHD (RESEARCH FOCUSED)
Approach	Implement change and evaluate: • Identify problems • Gather/critique research • Determine best practice • Implement solutions • Evaluate outcomes/process • Adopt/abandon practice • Repeat.	Scientific research methods: • Formulate a question • State hypothesis • Conduct an experiment or an observational study • Record/interpret findings • State the results • Share outcomes for potential use in practice • Repeat.

Source: Data from the American Association of Colleges of Nursing. (2021). *The essentials: Core competencies for professional nursing education.* https://www.aacnnursing.org/Education-Resources/AACN-Essentials; American Association of Colleges of Nursing. (2015). *The doctor of nursing practice: Current issues and clarifying recommendations* [White paper]. https://www.aacnnursing.org/Portals/42/News/White-Papers/DNP-Implementation-TF-Report-8-15.pdf; White, K. M., Dudley-Brown, S., & Terhaar, M. F. (Eds.). (2020). *Translation of evidence into nursing and healthcare* (3rd ed.). Springer Publishing Company.

In reviewing this information, write down at least two thoughts or questions you have for your faculty.

1.

2.

Reflection: DNP and PhD degrees. Dr. Melissa deCardi Hladek PhD, CRNP, FNP-BC, Johns Hopkins University.

The DNP and PhD degrees contribute to the nursing profession in distinct ways. It starts with purpose. If your purpose steers you to making a specific healthcare system or unit function more efficiently, the DNP degree may be the best fit for you. On the other hand, if you are interested in generating new knowledge or new systems of healthcare delivery, for example, the PhD may be a better fit. Your anticipated future role plays a part in this decision. Do you see yourself as primarily an advanced practice provider or nurse executive? The DNP degree may be best in that case. Rather, do you see yourself designing and conducting randomized control studies or qualitative studies? Those roles will lend themselves better to the PhD degree. Although both degrees involve components of research, the PhD will place greater emphasis with more extensive instruction and mentoring around research methodology, design, and analysis, whereas the DNP Project will emphasize a translational approach within a healthcare microsystem. The structures and duration of each program also differ. DNP coursework emphasizes leadership and advanced clinical skills, while the PhD structure involves coursework followed by extensive self-directed work on your area of inquiry. Both impact the nursing profession and the healthcare system to inform practice, policy, and education.

WHY DNP AND PHD? RACHEL RISNER, PHD, DNP, APRN, C-FNP, CNE

Students, colleagues, and friends have asked me repeatedly why I have two doctoral degrees. My answer is twofold, and my response is always the same. I completed my DNP degree first, as I felt it was important for me to complete a terminal degree that was clinically focused. I am a practicing family nurse practitioner. However, I work not only as a family nurse practitioner but also as a nurse educator in academia. So I felt it was equally important for me to complete my PhD in nursing education.

WHY DNP AND PHD? RACHEL RISNER, PHD, DNP, APRN, C-FNP, CNE

I learned so much wonderful information in both programs, but they were very different. The DNP program track that I completed was specifically designed for advanced practice nurses who already hold a master's degree in nursing and national certification as an advanced practice nurse. The program was not focused on gaining content that would allow me to specialize in a specific nursing role, but to provide coursework that assisted me in growing as a clinical leader and aided in developing the skills that I needed to effect positive change in the healthcare system. The DNP program helped me improve my critical thinking skills, evaluate evidence-based research, and to translate my knowledge into practice.

I enjoyed my DNP program immensely. But I wanted to develop my competency in research, so I applied for the PhD in the nursing education program. I felt strongly that I needed to complete this degree to be an expert in the field of nursing education. I was also acutely aware of the nurse faculty shortage that we are facing in the United States. My PhD program prepared me to be an expert nurse educator and researcher, which assists me in helping to advance nursing science. This program helped me develop skills in curriculum development, course evaluation, curriculum design, backward design, information technology, research, and theory development. This type of work is not the focus of a DNP program.

In my opinion, completing both degrees has been very beneficial in advancing my knowledge in research, clinical practice, and nursing education. Nurses with a DNP degree can be hired as faculty since it is a terminal degree. However, additional education-specific knowledge is needed beyond the DNP degree. I encourage you always to continue to learn and grow in your area of specialty. We can make positive changes in our healthcare systems by increasing our knowledge and understanding through furthering our education.

SHOULD I PURSUE A PHD OR DNP? WHERE IS THE VALUE? SALLIE PORTER, DNP, PHD, APN, RN-BC, CPNP

DNP students occasionally ask me why I chose to obtain both a DNP degree and a PhD degree. The answer is relatively simple: As a clinician, I wanted to hold the highest clinical practice degree available to me—the Doctor of Nursing Practice. I usually add that if the DNP degree had come along a bit sooner, that might have been my truly terminal degree.

However, what I learned as a PhD student (I got that degree first) certainly supported my learning as a DNP student. The PhD degree provided me with multiple research method courses, much more than I received in my DNP program, and a deeper understanding of data analysis (although I am still learning). My PhD gave me the time to develop my content expertise in a narrow area and gave me the flexibility to participate in three different fellowships during my time as a student. The opportunity to interact outside of your institution and learn with other professions provided a sound basis for much of what I do and value today. It also gave me plenty of opportunities to write—pretty much every assignment was to write a research-based paper or a research project. And to read—the required reading load was tremendous, especially for a person like me who worked full time. Overall, the PhD program really did help me learn to think differently and better.

My DNP degree program was more fast paced and was presented in a 3-day weekend model that met once a month. The model was designed to move you relatively quickly through the still-evolving DNP degree content. I already had my master's degree and post-master's pediatric nurse practitioner certification, so the content was strictly DNP degree content and not the role content that many students are trying to master as well in a BSN-to-DNP degree program. I cannot emphasize enough what a challenge it can be to learn a new role as part of a doctoral degree. New things I learned in the DNP degree program included a systematic review as a method, that many PhD nurses did not truly understand the DNP degree, the struggles of group work, and how important understanding your stakeholders and setting are to implementing change. Overall, the DNP degree provided me with the information needed to take knowledge and implement it in a way to improve health outcomes.

> **SHOULD I PURSUE A PHD OR DNP? WHERE IS THE VALUE? SALLIE PORTER, DNP, PHD, APN, RN-BC, CPNP**
>
> As evidenced by the sheer numbers of nurses working to obtain their DNP degree and the plethora of new and planned DNP programs, I would say that nurses have voted with their feet and the DNP degree won! Of course, we still do need nurse scientists. We need DNP-educated nurses to further assume leadership positions in healthcare institutions, professional associations, schools of nursing, and governmental and health policy agencies. We also need to ensure that DNP-educated nurses determine what the degree encapsulates and how best to process learners to that end point. The DNP may be a terminal degree, but for nurses, patients, and healthcare providers, it is just the beginning of a wonderful journey that I believe will ultimately change healthcare for the better.

SUMMARY

The DNP is a practice-focused degree with an emphasis on implementing and evaluating changes in the healthcare setting. The PhD is a research-focused degree centered on more traditional concepts of science. In the next lesson, we will further explore the elements of the DNP Project.

NEXT STEPS

- Continue to explore the distinguishing features of both the DNP and the PhD to promote future collaboration by reading the article by Murphy et al. (2015) in "References and Resources."
- Talk to your faculty if you have questions.

REFERENCES AND RESOURCES

American Association of Colleges of Nursing. (2006). *DNP essentials*. https://www.aacnnursing.org/DNP/DNP-Essentials

American Association of Colleges of Nursing. (2015). *The doctor of nursing practice: Current issues and clarifying recommendations*. https://www.aacnnursing.org/Portals/42/DNP/DNP-Implementation.pdf

American Association of Colleges of Nursing. (2021). *The essentials: Core competencies for professional nursing education*. https://www.aacnnursing.org/Education-Resources/AACN-Essentials

Murphy, M., Stafflieno, B., & Carlson, E. (2015). Collaboration among DNP- and PhD-prepared nurses. *Journal of Professional Nursing*, 31(5), 388–394. https://doi.org/10.1016/j.profnurs.2015.03.001

White, K. M., Dudley-Brown, S., & Terhaar, M. F (Eds.). (2020). *Translation of evidence into nursing and healthcare* (3rd ed.). Springer Publishing Company.

RELATED TEXTBOOK

White, K. M., Dudley-Brown, S., & Terhaar, M. F (Eds.). (2020). *Translation of evidence into nursing and healthcare* (3rd ed.). Springer Publishing Company.

LESSON 2.5

EVIDENCE-BASED PRACTICE AND QUALITY IMPROVEMENT

BACKGROUND

All nurses should be committed to the idea of using the best information available to make the best decisions they can for their patients. The term "evidence-based practice (EBP)" is defined as "the conscientious, explicit, and judicious use of the integration of current best evidence, clinical expertise, and patient values into the decision-making process for patient care" (Christenbery, 2018, p. 5). Although good in theory, use of evidence in clinical practice can be difficult. Because the implementation of EBP may be difficult, there is a reluctance to change the status quo. However, to provide high-quality, evidence-based care for patients, we must be vigilant to optimize care through proven methods.

The Institute for Healthcare Improvement (IHI) states that the goal should be to improve the health of patient populations by providing access to quality care at affordable costs (IHI, 2018). This has been coined "The Triple Aim." If we include the self-care of the healthcare team, this is referred to as "The Quadruple Aim" (Figure 2.2).

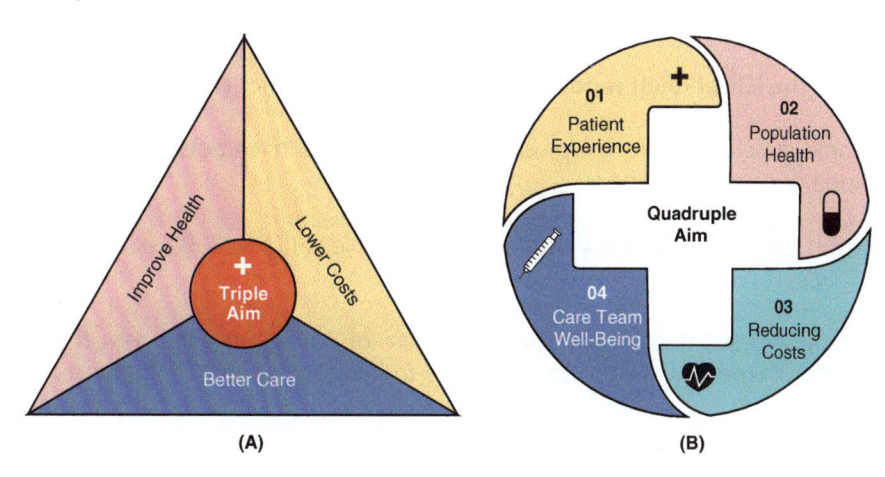

Figure 2.2 (A) The Triple Aim. (B) The Quadruple Aim.

Florence Nightingale used evidence to improve the quality of nursing care. The modern momentum to improve quality in healthcare is well articulated in a series of documents published by the Institute of Medicine (IOM), *To Err Is Human* in 1999, *Crossing the Quality Chasm* in 2001, and *The Future of Nursing* report (IOM, 2011). These are landmark documents that every DNP student must read and carefully review in detail. The links to the document summaries are provided here

- 1999: *To Err Is Human* (https://www.nap.edu/read/9728/chapter/1)
- 2001: *Crossing the Quality Chasm* (https://www.nap.edu/catalog/10027/crossing-the-quality-chasm-a-new-health-system-for-the)
- 2011: *The Future of Nursing: Leading Change, Advancing Health* (https://www.nap.edu/read/12956/chapter/1)

These documents highlight the gaps in healthcare and the need for continuous quality improvement. Unacceptably, people entering the healthcare system are harmed by *preventable* oversights and/or errors.

The IOM landmark reports (IOM, 1999, 2001) reveal variations in cost and quality of care, thus negatively impacting outcomes.

In a follow-up report to the 2001 *Crossing the Quality Chasm* report, the IOM released *Health Professions Education: A Bridge to Quality*, which states that health professional education programs should include competencies in five areas: (a) patient-centered care, (b) quality improvement, (c) interprofessional collaborative practice, (d) health information technology, and (e) EBP (IOM, 2003). When you align the publication of these documents with the origins of the DNP degree in the early 2000s, it is clear to see the relationship between competency-based education and the need for continuous evaluation of outcomes to assess for gaps in care and to implement necessary improvements. Nurses with a practice focus need a higher level of skill and education to be change agents in the modern healthcare environment. Experiences to engage and develop greater familiarity with EBP for quality improvement and assurance are necessary.

LEARNING OBJECTIVES

- Examine the IOM documents: *To Err Is Human, Crossing the Quality Chasm,* and *A Bridge to Quality.*
- Define the qualities of "good" healthcare.
- Compare and discuss the features of three process models:
  - The steps of the EBP process
  - IHI: Model for Improvement
  - The scientific method

ACTIVITIES

Use the summary of the IOM (1999) report, *To Err Is Human,* to extract these key points:

At least 44,000 people die annually from a medical error that could have been prevented (IOM, 1999). What are some of the types of errors that occur?

According to the report, errors are not really caused by "bad apples" (IOM, 2001, p. 2), but are more commonly caused by what?

A goal set was to reduce preventable errors by a minimum of 50% within the next 5 years. To achieve this goal, a strategy for improvement was described, using a four-tiered approach. What are those four tiers?

1. _____
2. _____
3. _____
4. _____

Read the summary of the IOM (2001) report, *Crossing the Quality Chasm*. This document outlines six specific attributes of "good" or "quality" healthcare. Use the document to describe the intended meaning:

Safe:

Effective:

Patient centered:

Timely:

Efficient:

Equitable:

☑ **If the healthcare system were to be redesigned, what are some general principles to use? There are 10 rules for redesign listed in the IOM (2001) report, *Crossing the Quality Chasm*.**

☑ **Based on your clinical practice today, do you think quality is being achieved? Is there room for improvement?**

☑ **There are many models and frameworks for making changes and improving the quality of healthcare. It is important to note that both a DNP- and a PhD-prepared nurse can make improvements in healthcare, yet the approach differs. The DNP-prepared nurse is more likely to use models and frameworks rooted in EBP and quality improvement (QI; see Figure 2.3). The PhD-prepared nurse develops new knowledge for the science of nursing, thus utilizing a scientific method (see Figure 2.5). Refer to each model (Figures 2.3–2.5) and read the supplemental materials. How do these frameworks compare and how do they contrast?**

- What are we trying to accomplish?
- How will we know that a change is an improvement?
- What change can we make that will result in improvement?

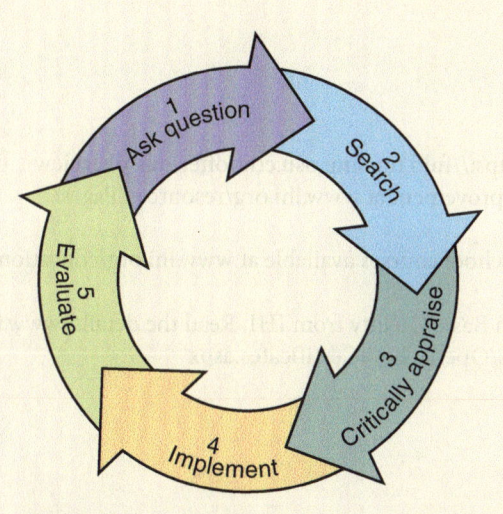

Figure 2.3 The steps of the evidence-based practice process.

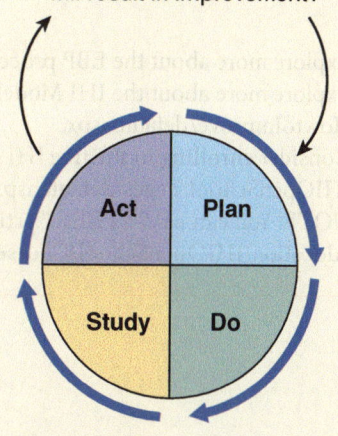

Figure 2.4 Model for Improvement.

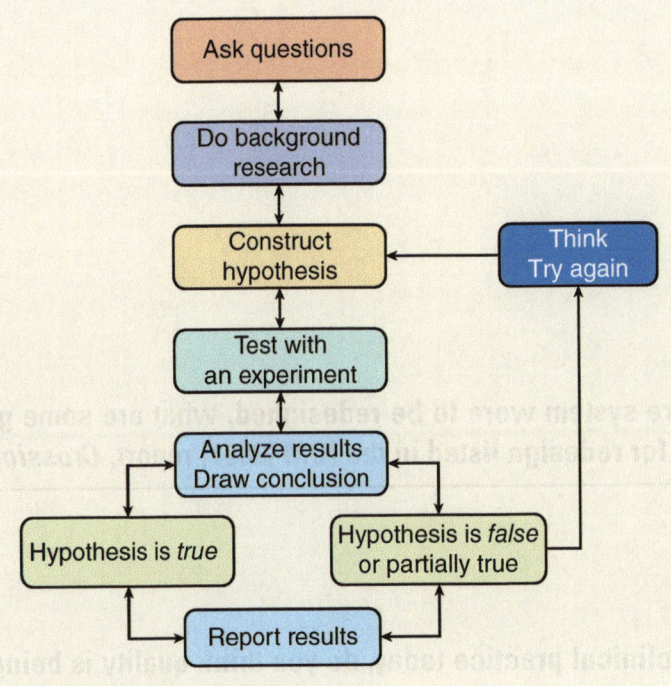

Figure 2.5 Scientific method.
Source: Reproduced with permission from Langley, G. J., Moen, R. D., Nolan, K. M., Nolan, T. W., Norman, C. L., & Provost, L. P. (2009). *The improvement guide: A practical approach to enhancing organizational performance.* Jossey-Bass.

SUMMARY

The DNP Project is an academic experience designed to help prepare nurses to lead changes at the highest level in the practice setting, which will improve the quality of healthcare (AACN, 2006, 2015). The DNP Project is rooted in concepts of EBP and QI. It borrows concepts and terminology from science and research, but does not fully embrace the precise rigor of the scientific method, as it has a different purpose.

NEXT STEPS

- Explore more about the EBP process at https://fuld.nursing.osu.edu/offerings-overview
- Explore more about the IHI Model for Improvement at www.ihi.org/resources/Pages/HowtoImprove/default.aspx
- Consider enrolling in the free IHI Open School courses available at www.ihi.org/education/IHIOpenSchool/Pages/default.aspx
- NOTE: You can earn a FREE Certificate in Basic Quality from IHI. Read the details: www.ihi.org/education/IHIOpenSchool/Courses/Pages/OpenSchoolCertificates.aspx

REFERENCES AND RESOURCES

Agency for Healthcare Research and Quality. (2008). *Six domains of quality in healthcare.* https://www.ahrq.gov/talkingquality/measures/six-domains.html

American Association of Colleges of Nursing. (2006). *The essentials of doctoral education for advanced nursing practice.* https://www.aacnnursing.org/Portals/42/Publications/DNPEssentials.pdf

American Association of Colleges of Nursing. (2015). *The doctor of nursing practice: Current issues and clarifying recommendations.* [White paper]. https://www.aacnnursing.org/Portals/42/News/White-Papers/DNP-Implementation-TF-Report-8-15.pdf

Berwick, D., & Whittington, J. (2008). The triple aim: Care, health, and cost. *Health Affairs, 27*(3), 759–769. https://doi.org/10.1377/hlthaff.27.3.759

Institute for Healthcare Improvement. (2018). *Science of improvement.* http://www.ihi.org/about/Pages/ScienceofImprovement.aspx

Institute of Medicine. (1999). *To err is human: Building a safer healthcare system, summary.* http://www.nationalacademies.org/hmd/~/media/Files/Report%20Files/1999/To-Err-is-Human/To%20Err%20is%20Human%201999%20%20report%20brief.pdf

Institute of Medicine. (2001). *Crossing the quality chasm, summary.* http://www.nationalacademies.org/hmd/~/media/Files/Report%20Files/2001/Crossing-the-Quality-Chasm/Quality%20Chasm%202001%20%20report%20brief.pdf

Institute of Medicine. (2003). *Health professions education: A bridge to quality.* National Academies Press. http://www.nationalacademies.org/hmd/Reports/2003/Health-Professions-Education-A-Bridge-to-Quality.aspx

Institute of Medicine. (2011). *The future of nursing: Leading change, advancing health.* National Academies Press.

Langley, G. J., Moen, R. D., Nolan, K. M., Nolan, T. W., Norman, C. L., & Provost, L. P. (2009). *The improvement guide: A practical approach to enhancing organizational performance.* Jossey-Bass.

RELATED TEXTBOOKS

Christenbery, T (Ed.). (2018). *Evidence-based practice in nursing.* Springer Publishing Company.

Hickey, J. V., & Brosnan, C. A (Eds.). (2017). *Evaluation of health care quality for DNPs* (2nd ed.). Springer Publishing Company.

LESSON 2.6

WHAT IS A DNP PROJECT?

BACKGROUND

The DNP is a practice-focused degree to prepare nurse leaders at the highest level of nursing practice to translate research, improve patient outcomes, and transform healthcare (American Association of Colleges of Nursing [AACN], 2015, 2023). The application and translation of evidence into practice are pivotal aspects of the DNP Project. The DNP Project demonstrates clinical scholarship and includes three specific components for all students: planning, implementation, and evaluation (AACN, 2023). The *Essentials* (AACN, 2021) provides a foundational framework for competency-based education. A DNP Project is the scholarly work for students to demonstrate attainment of entry-level and advanced-level competencies, along with the advanced specialty/role competencies (AACN, 2021).

Students seeking a practice doctorate in nursing are required to complete scholarly work that aims to improve clinical outcome (AACN, 2021). The DNP Project is intended as an opportunity for students to expand knowledge, integrate new skills into practice, and demonstrate competencies and principles of nursing scholarship (AACN, 2023). Healthcare is dynamic and necessitates a transformative and innovative perspective. The nature of the DNP Project continues to evolve and is dynamic, thus supporting the transitions in healthcare. Therefore, DNP students and graduates have great potential to impact system-level outcomes by translating evidence into practice and health policy (AACN, 2022). By completing a scholarly DNP Project, the student becomes equipped with high-level problem-solving skills to lead and engage in evidence-based projects well beyond graduation.

The intended purpose of the DNP Project is to promote a solution to a micro-, meso-, or macro-level systems gap in practice (AACN, 2023). The requirements and elements of the project vary based on the nurse's role, partnering agency, university requirements, and other variables. At some universities, the DNP Project was initially modeled after a PhD dissertation. Some schools initially used a portfolio model in which students collected work from different courses to complete a final product. There are varying perspectives on the utilization of group projects. Nonetheless, integrative or systematic reviews as a final project alone are not considered a DNP Project (AACN, 2015, 2023).

In 2022, the State of the DNP Summary Report (AACN, 2022) identified the overall goal for the DNP Project is to improve quality and patient outcomes, as well as achieve practice change. However, there is variability with the implementation process among DNP programs (AACN, 2022). Previously, AACN (2015) published a white paper titled, "The Doctor of Nursing Practice: Current Issues and Clarifying Recommendations." This paper sought to describe and define the DNP Project expectations and remains a pivotal reference. Additionally, the AACN (2023) provided a DNP Project Toolkit for information and as a resource to inform the scholarly project (explore this website at https://www.aacnnursing.org/our-initiatives/education-practice/doctor-of-nursing-practice/tool-kit). These resources collectively can provide foundational information to inform the DNP Project.

In this lesson, we will explore AACN resources to establish a baseline for your DNP Project. In subsequent lessons, incorporation of expectations regarding your university and guidance are offered for additional project considerations.

LEARNING OBJECTIVES

- Read the AACN's (2015) "The Doctor of Nursing Practice: Current Issues and Clarifying Recommendations."
- Explore the DNP Toolkit (AACN, 2023).
- Extrapolate elements of the resources to inform your DNP Project.

ACTIVITIES

Use the AACN (2015) document to extract and outline key information. We help you dissect the meaning of the sections as you work.

Section II. The DNP Project, p. 3. Complete this sentence.

Title: "The final scholarly project should be called _____."

Learning Point: The scholarly project is not referred to as a "capstone project." The word "capstone" is confusing due to the use in undergraduate nursing curriculum and in other professions. It is also not "research" or a "dissertation," as these terms are aligned with a PhD degree. The DNP degree utilizes the term "DNP Project" to represent scholarly work.

Section II. The DNP Project, p. 4. Complete these sentences.

Scholarly Product: "The elements of the DNP Project should be the same for all students and include planning, implementation, and evaluation components. . . . All DNP Projects should:

a. Focus on a change _____.
b. Have a system or _____."
c. Demonstrate _____.
d. Include a plan for _____.
e. Include an evaluation of _____.
f. Provide a foundation for _____.

Learning Point: These are minimum expectations of the DNP Project. Some projects may be more robust in terms of one element compared to others.

Section II. The DNP Project, p. 5. Complete this sentence.

Dissemination of the DNP Project should include _____.

Learning Point: Dissemination is a vital component to the profession of nursing. As colleagues, we learn from one another. It is important to share your DNP Project to a broader audience. Colleagues may want to implement something similar in their work setting. The public may benefit from some part of the information. Remember at the highest levels of practice and scholarship, it is often necessary to share information in different ways depending on the audience. Outcomes from your DNP Project should be disseminated in multiple ways, including a final academic paper, a final presentation to stakeholders, and a final poster or presentation at a regional, state, national, or international conference. Review the DNP Project Toolkit for additional suggestions and guidelines. The requirements for your university will be reviewed later in the workbook.

Section II. The DNP Project, p. 5. Take notice and investigate.

The AACN recommends the use of a digital repository to catalog and share DNP Projects. Most academic institutions have a repository available and require doctoral students to use them (inquire at your academic institution). Independent repositories are available. Keenly review the organizational policies on their use and requirements for de-identification of sensitive project information. Here are the links to some repositories for you to explore:

- The Virginia Henderson Library: www.nursingrepository.org/
- Doctors of Nursing Practice, Inc.: https://www.doctorsofnursingpractice.org/doctoral-project-repository/
- Emory University: https://etd.library.emory.edu/
- Johns Hopkins University: https://nursing.jhu.edu/academics/programs/doctoral/dnp/capstone.html
- Ohio State University: https://kb.osu.edu/handle/1811/48671
- University of San Francisco: https://repository.usfca.edu/dnp/
- University of Massachusetts Amherst: https://scholarworks.umass.edu/nursing_dnp_capstone/

- University of Pennsylvania: https://repository.upenn.edu/dnp_projects/
- University of Texas at San Antonio: http://library.uthscsa.edu/2011/09/etd/

Section II. The DNP Project, p. 5. Answer the following question.

DNP Project team: Why should the term "DNP Project team" be used instead of "committee"?

Answer: _____

Learning Point: The DNP Project process differs from the PhD dissertation process.

SUMMARY

You have now been introduced to the minimum expectations of a DNP Project as outlined by the AACN. In a future lesson plan, the requirements at your university will be explored. As the chapter concludes, we continue to refer to the AACN documents to inform and clarify other project-related concepts such as the types of project, considerations for group projects, the DNP practice experience, and the DNP practice hours. In the next lesson plan, you will be introduced to types of DNP Projects.

NEXT STEPS

- Obtain the DNP Project requirements at your university.
- Read and reflect on how they relate to what you have learned in this lesson.

REFERENCES AND RESOURCES

American Association of Colleges of Nursing. (2006). *The essentials of doctoral education for advanced nursing practice.* https://www.aacnnursing.org/Portals/42/Publications/DNPEssentials.pdf

American Association of Colleges of Nursing. (2015). *The doctor of nursing practice: Current issues and clarifying recommendations.* https://www.aacnnursing.org/Portals/42/DNP/DNP-Implementation.pdf

American Association of Colleges of Nursing. (2021). *The essentials: Core competencies for professional nursing education.* https://www.aacnnursing.org/Education-Resources/AACN-Essentials

American Association of Colleges of Nursing. (2022). *The state of doctor of nursing practice education in 2022.* https://www.aacnnursing.org/Portals/42/News/Surveys-Data/State-of-the-DNP-Summary-Report-June-2022.pdf

American Association of Colleges of Nursing. (2023). *Doctor of nursing practice (DNP) tool kit.* https://www.aacnnursing.org/our-initiatives/education-practice/doctor-of-nursing-practice/tool-kit

Institute of Medicine. (2011). *The future of nursing: Leading change, advancing health.* National Academies Press.

RELATED TEXTBOOK

Christenbery, T (Ed.). (2018). *Evidence-based practice in nursing.* Springer Publishing Company.
  Unit II: Designing and Implementing Evidence-Based Practice Projects

LESSON 2.7

DESIGN TYPES OF DNP PROJECTS

BACKGROUND

The purpose of the DNP Project is to focus on a change that impacts healthcare outcomes for patients, systems, and communities, which demonstrates a student's scholarly work during their DNP program. The goal of the DNP Project is to translate current best evidence to improve the quality of healthcare, outcomes, and systems, involving a process that includes a project design, implementation (direct or nondirect), evaluation, and dissemination (American Association of Colleges of Nursing [AACN], 2021; Hinch et al., 2020). The DNP Project design types share many universal elements, such as the DNP Team, Approach, and Intention of the components. Additionally, the DNP Project's ultimate goal is to improve the health of patient populations, either directly or indirectly, aligning with the *Essentials* (AACN, 2021) and the Institute for Healthcare Improvement's (IHI, 2018) "The Triple Aim" and "The Quadruple Aim" (Figure 2.2). As highlighted in Lesson 2.4, the DNP Project includes problem identification; an expansive review of literature, analysis, and synthesis; translating evidence to construct a strategy or method to address a problem; designing an implementation plan and actual implementation; and the evaluation of outcomes, processes, and/or experience (AACN, 2021).

The DNP Project is the cultivation and the cornerstone of scholarly practice work occurring during a DNP program, is often a graduation requirement, and contributes to launching a doctoral-prepared nurse's scholarly trajectory after graduation (AACN, 2022). The DNP Project, including the former names that have been used (i.e., "Capstone Project"), have evolved over time since the inception of the DNP degree, beginning when two instrumental agencies formed a collaborative relationship defining the DNP degree and what entails a rigorous DNP Project, the AACN and the National Organization of Nurse Practitioner Faculties (NONPF; AACN, 2004). To better gauge the evolution, trends, and utilization of DNP-prepared nurses' practice and roles, the AACN conducted a study in 2020 examining DNP graduates that identified seven recommendations, including clarifying the rigor and types of DNP Projects (AACN, 2022). There has been a plethora of recent literature outlining ideal project processes and types of DNP Projects that align with the *Essentials* (AACN, 2021) and the NONPF Core Competencies (2022).

LEARNING OBJECTIVES

- Review the background of the evolution of DNP Projects.
- Discuss the key national and nursing agencies that influence the types of commonly used DNP Projects.
- Summarize commonly used DNP Project designs' purpose and intent, and review nomenclature, methodology, framework examples, and resources.
- Explore your own project's possible design and discuss with faculty and colleagues.

Choosing a Design Type

When choosing a DNP Project type, the priority is congruence of many factors to identify an appropriate format that aligns with the clinical problem occurring at the organizational site, the population of interest, and the strategic goals (outcomes) that will lead to an improvement in healthcare delivery. The DNP student must perform a "background" assessment of these noted variables and develop an understanding and relationship with the stakeholders of the organizational site to build a strong foundation for the DNP Project. Preparation includes searching the evidence in the literature and developing an evidence synthesis of the noted clinical problem and identifying evidence-based "solutions." This formative work will guide the student in determining the appropriate type of DNP Project for that particular problem, site/setting, stakeholders, involved healthcare professionals, projected/proposed outcomes and goals, data methodology plan, and the target population, system, or community needs and feasibility. The clinical question of inquiry will develop from this formative process, also guiding the student in determining the appropriate congruent project design type. It is crucial to clarify that the type of possible intervention (implementation activities) identified in the evidence search should not guide the project type choice. There is no *"one size fits all"* when determining a project type (design) to develop; many facets and factors must be identified and critically reviewed prior to determining the "best project type fit."

Common Types of DNP Project Designs

There are a variety of DNP Project designs that can be utilized and driven by the identified problem, associated factors noted previously, and the developed clinical question. It is equally important to note that DNP Projects are not meant to be experimental, novel, hypothesis testing, or generalizable in design. This style of research is predominantly conducted by PhD nurse scientists (see PhD vs. DNP lesson). The most common DNP Project design types include Quality Improvement (QI)/Process Improvement (PI), Evidence-Based Practice (EBP), Health/Legislative Policy, and Program Development and Evaluation (PD/PE). The following table highlights commonly used project design types. Although there may be the occasional rare need to consider alternative design types to meet the needs of the population of interest, project site, and nature of the healthcare problem identified (Table 2.1).

Table 2.1 Common DNP Project Design Types

DESIGN TYPES	PURPOSE AND INTENT	METHODOLOGICAL APPROACH/FRAMEWORK EXAMPLES
QI/Process/PI	A systematic approach to understanding and identifying EBP/best-practice approach, often using a PICO question to guide an internal evidence search (and external when indicated), that will lead to improved population healthcare outcomes (improvement of the problem) by test-implementing or improving usage of proven strategies, protocols, processes, or interventions and then evaluating the problem's outcome change in a specific healthcare setting/site and population group (IHI, 2018; Melnyk & Fineout-Overholt, 2023).	IHI Model for Improvement, PDSA Cycle (IHI, 2018)
EBP	To identify the best scientific evidence (EBP) via a thorough external systematic search and critical appraisal (PICO or question of inquiry) combined with clinical expertise and population or systems' circumstances (via fishbone or concept map) to make informed healthcare decisions to answer a clinical inquiry that facilitates the Quadruple Aims (IHI, 2018; Melnyk & Fineout-Overholt, 2023)	The Seven Steps of the EBP Process (Melnyk & Fineout-Overholt, 2023) JH EBP Model (Dang et al., 2021).

(continued)

DESIGN TYPES	PURPOSE AND INTENT	METHODOLOGICAL APPROACH/FRAMEWORK EXAMPLES
EBQI	Applying the EBP problem-solving approach to a QI project (see earlier). The goal of QI should be that it is a best-practice/EBP-driven rigorous systematic search of internal (via fishbone or concept map) and external evidence with the best available experiential evidence to deliberately guide informed decision-making and identify the best approach to improve the clinical problem at the site and incorporate population or systems-specific circumstances (Dang et al., 2021).	JH EBP Model (Dang et al., 2021).
Health/ Legislative Policy Analyses	A systematic interdisciplinary approach and collaboration to identifying, analyzing, and prioritizing policy/legislation (such as a root-cause analysis) that can improve population or systems' healthcare outcomes in order to address public health problems and analyze policies/legislation to understand their potential health impact on populations and economic impact by identifying evidence-based policy solutions, advocacy, and gaps occurring at the agency, state, national, or global levels (CDC, 2023a). The process of policy development should be a systematic and planned approach, such as using the Yoder-Wise, which incorporates four major filters that are key considerations and behaviors that will ensure the integrity of the policy being analyzed, reviewed, or developed (2020).	CDC's Policy Analytical Framework (2013) Yoder-Wise Framework for Planned Policy Change (2020)
PD/PE	An intent-driven interdisciplinary systematic study (root-cause analyses), evaluation, and proposal of a healthcare program's processes and outcomes to evaluate the need for further program development, modifications, intervention strategies, or revisions to improve the effectiveness and sustainability of a specific healthcare program; the proposal involves methods that are useful, feasible, ethical, sustainable, and accurate with the overarching goal of improved healthcare outcomes for a specific site and population of interest (CDC, 2023).	Centers for Disease Control and Prevention. Framework for program evaluation in public health. MMWR 1999;48 (No. RR-11)

CDC, Centers for Disease Control and Prevention; EBP, evidence-based practice; EBQI, evidence-based quality improvement; IHI, Institute for Healthcare Improvement; PD/PE, Program Development and Evaluation; PDSA, Plan-Do-Study-Act; PI, protocol improvement; PICO, patient/problem, intervention, comparison, outcome; QI, quality improvement.

Sources: Centers for Disease Control and Prevention. (1999). *Framework for program evaluation in public health*. https://www.cdc.gov/evaluation/framework/index.htm; Centers for Disease Control and Prevention. (2013). *CDC's policy analytical framework*. https://www.cdc.gov/policy/paeo/process/analysis.html; Centers for Disease Control and Prevention. (2023). *A framework for program evaluation*. https://www.cdc.gov/evaluation/framework/index.htm#:~:text=A%20Framework%20for%20Program%20Evaluation&text=The%20Framework%20for%20Evaluation%20in,essential%20elements%20of%20program%20evaluation; Dang, D., Dearhold, S. L., Bissett, K., Ascenzi, J., & Whalen, M. (2021). *Johns Hopkins evidence-based practice for nurses and healthcare professionals: Model & guidelines'* (4th ed.). Sigma Theta Tau; Institute for Healthcare Improvement. (2018). *Science of improvement*. https://www.ihi.org/resources/how-to-improve; Melnyk, B. M., & Fineout-Overholt, E. (2023). *Evidence-based practice in nursing and healthcare: A guide to best practice* (5th ed.). Wolters Kluwer; Yoder-Wise, P. S. (2020). *A framework for planned policy change. Nursing Forum, 55*(1), 45–53. https://doi.org/10.1111/nuf.12381.

ACTIVITY

Reviewing the background of the evolution of DNP Projects and common design types is an essential step along your DNP Project development journey. It is wise not to rush this process and to take into account project considerations, as in a "who, what, where, and how" approach; these include:

- Who: who are the affected populations of interest?
- What: the specificities of the clinical problem (first and foremost) and what does the evidence "tell" you?
- Where: identify the needs of the project site (site justification), agency (strategic goals/priorities), program, and/or policy/legislation and how does this intersect with the problem (root-cause analyses, fishbone, and/or concept map analyses) to improve the identified healthcare problem?
- How: consider and evaluate your DNP Project team and stakeholder support, and evaluate the feasibility, sustainability, timeline, and financial aspects of the project you are considering; is this project "doable"?

Partner with a colleague and discuss each other's projects and answer the following questions:

1. Based on the types of DNP Project designs, what have you learned?
    1.
    2.
    3.
2. Considering your possible "who, what, where, and how" of your project, which type of project is best suited?
3. Provide the rationale and references; which methodological framework is best suited for your project's design?
4. What questions do you still have?
    1.
    2.
    3.

REFERENCES AND RESOURCES

American Association of Colleges of Nursing. (2004). *AACN position statement on the practice doctorate in nursing.* https://www.aacnnursing.org/Portals/42/News/Position-Statements/DNP.pdf

American Association of Colleges of Nursing. (2021). *The essentials: Core competencies for professional nursing education.* https://www.aacnnursing.org/Education-Resources/AACN-Essentials

American Association of Colleges of Nursing. (2022). *The state of doctor of nursing practice education in 2022.* https://www.aacnnursing.org/Portals/42/News/Surveys-Data/State-of-the-DNP-Summary-Report-June-2022.pdf

Hinch, B. K., Livesay, S., Stifter, J., & Brown, Jr., F. (2020). Academic-practice partnerships: Building a sustainable model for doctor of nursing practice (DNP) projects. *Journal of Professional Nursing, 36*(6), 569–578.v

Institute for Healthcare Improvement. (2018). *Science of improvement.* http://www.ihi.org/about/Pages/ScienceofImprovement.aspx

National Organization of Nurse Practitioner Faculties. (2022). *National organization of nurse practitioner faculties' nurse practitioner role core competencies.* https://www.nonpf.org/page/14

LESSON 2.8

DNP PROJECT REQUIREMENTS AT YOUR SCHOOL

BACKGROUND

The minimum expectations for DNP Projects are informed by the *Essentials* (American Association of Colleges of Nursing [AACN], 2021) and further clarified by the AACN report, "The Doctor of Nursing Practice: Current Issues and Clarifying Recommendations" (AACN, 2015). The individual school or university further outlines its expectations for DNP Projects.

LEARNING OBJECTIVES

- Outline the DNP Project requirements at your school.
- Review the expected AACN requirements for the DNP Project and compare with your academic institution project requirements.
- List questions to address or clarify with your faculty or mentor.

ACTIVITIES

It is your responsibility as a student to understand the DNP Project requirements at your academic institution. The following questions help you to identify and organize pertinent information. Make a list of questions to further clarify with your faculty or mentor.

Do you have the most current version of the academic institution's DNP Project requirements? _____

Who is your academic advisor or project advisor? _____

What is their contact information? _____

What is their role for your DNP Project? _____

What type of DNP degree program are you enrolled in? _____

What is your anticipated date of graduation? _____

☑ **Take some notes. In reviewing this information, how does the DNP Project process work at your academic institution? Here are some key points to consider.**

- How is the topic for the DNP Project identified?
- At what point in your curriculum does a topic need to be solidified?
- Who determines where, or in what context, the DNP Project will be implemented?
- What is the process for creating the DNP Project Team?
- What are the requirements for the DNP Team members for your academic institution?
- What types of DNP Projects are permitted or have been completed at your school?
- Does the school permit group projects? If so, how does the process work?
- How is the DNP Project proposal developed and approved? Is there a dedicated course within the curriculum or the DNP Project completed outside of coursework?
- Does the academic institution require memorandum of understanding (MOU) for DNP Projects to be completed?
- How does the student identify and collaboratively work with agencies and other project stakeholders?
- Does the academic institution offer support for project-related scholarly writing and statistics?
- What are the requirements of the DNP Project including the development of a paper, presentation, and dissemination of findings?
- Does the school provide a guide for you to follow?

Questions for Faculty or Mentor

_____
_____
_____
_____
_____
_____

SUMMARY

Along your journey to complete your DNP Project, there will be many questions. Keep a running list of your questions to discuss with your faculty or mentor. It is common to feel overwhelmed at this point, yet rest assured there are supports. In this lesson, you have discovered the DNP Project requirements at your academic institution. Being prepared and equipped with an understanding of the requirements provides an easier path.

In the next lesson, you will review actual DNP Projects. By reviewing some final products, you gain an understanding of what is expected.

NEXT STEPS

- Access two published DNP Projects from your academic institution and review for the next activity.
- If access is limited, utilize online repositories listed previously to select projects to review. Your faculty may assign projects for the class to review for later discussion.

REFERENCES AND RESOURCES

American Association of Colleges of Nursing. (2015). *The doctor of nursing practice: Current issues and clarifying recommendations*. https://www.aacnnursing.org/Portals/42/DNP/DNP-Implementation.pdf

American Association of Colleges of Nursing. (2021). *The essentials: Core competencies for professional nursing education*. https://www.aacnnursing.org/Education-Resources/AACN-Essentials

American Association of Colleges of Nursing. (2023). *Doctor of nursing practice (DNP) tool kit*. https://www.aacnnursing.org/our-initiatives/education-practice/doctor-of-nursing-practice/tool-kit

Below are some examples of DNP Project requirements from various universities:

Emory University. (2023). *Doctor of nursing practice program handbook*. https://assets-global.website-files.com/5f11b12012400490893a64ea/63bc6276291a4c60403393ee_DNP%20Handbook%20Final%202022-2023%20(Fall%202022).pdf

Purdue University. (2022). *Doctor of nursing practice: Practice inquiry project guidelines and checklist. Author*. https://www.pnw.edu/college-of-nursing/wp-content/uploads/sites/82/2020/10/DNPProjectChecklist09.21.20.docx

Rush University College of Nursing. (2018). *Doctor of nursing practice program project guide*. https://www.rushu.rush.edu/sites/default/files/College%20of%20Nursing/Rush%20DNP%20Project%20Guide.pdf

Rutgers School of Nursing. (n.d.). *DNP toolkit*. https://nursing.rutgers.edu/students/dnp-toolkit/

LESSON 2.9

REVIEW OF COMPLETED DNP PROJECTS

BACKGROUND

It is important to examine exemplars of completed projects as you begin your DNP journey. When looking at previous student projects, it can be easier to see a product in its final format. Most academic institutions have an online repository of previous projects for potential and incoming students to view.

In this lesson, select two complete projects from your school to review, if possible. The chapter also has links to completed projects for your review. The goal is to see how DNP Projects are developed based on what we have learned. We will use the minimum expectations published by the American Association of Colleges of Nursing (AACN, 2021) to guide our discussion.

The objective is not to categorize the projects in this review as "good projects" or as "bad projects." The projects selected have something to offer to spark conversation and promote learning. Selected projects can be freely accessed, in full, online. Topics were selected to represent subjects that can be generalized to most topics in clinical nursing.

There is no "perfect" DNP Project. When a DNP project is reviewed, there may be identifiable areas that need improvement; however, there are a plethora of completed DNP Projects. There are many approaches to take when conducting a DNP project, and each offers knowledge in their own way. The DNP Project offers a learning experience. You are experiencing a growth process, and after graduation, the goal is to continue to translate best evidence into practice. The knowledge and skills you acquire while completing your DNP program and project serve as a foundation for further scholarship.

LEARNING OBJECTIVES

- Inventory select elements of completed DNP Projects.
- Summarize observations and discuss them with classmates and faculty.

ACTIVITIES

Read the following completed DNP Projects. Take notes as you identify the DNP Project expectations described by AACN (2023). (Editable versions of these activities may be accessed at connect.springerpub.com/content/book/978-0-8261-7484-0/chapter/ch02.)

DNP PROJECT REVIEW I

Project Title: "The 5A's Model for Smoking Cessation: Engaging Health Care Providers and Overcoming Barriers to Change." Retrieved from https://sigma.nursingrepository.org/handle/10755/620614

AACN PROJECT ELEMENTS	REVIEW NOTES
What was "changed" in practice and how did it impact healthcare outcomes?	
Was there a focus on a population or system? Explain.	
How did the project demonstrate implementation? What was done?	
What outcomes or processes were evaluated?	
How was practice or policy impacted by the project?	
How will the project be sustained?	
Were plans for future scholarship discussed?	

DNP PROJECT REVIEW II

Project Title: "Standardizing Smoking Cessation Intervention for Patients in an Acute Care Setting" (The full project write-up by Michelle Santoro is available via Springer Publishing Connect™. Access the supplement via connect.springerpub.com/content/book/978-0-8261-7484-0/chapter/ch02 and select the "Show additional chapter resources" button.)

AACN PROJECT ELEMENTS	REVIEW NOTES
What was "changed" in practice and how did it impact healthcare outcomes?	
Was there a focus on a population or system? Explain.	
How did the project demonstrate implementation? What was done?	
What outcomes or processes were evaluated?	
How was practice or policy impacted by the project?	
How will the project be sustained?	
Were plans for future scholarship discussed?	

How are the two projects similar and how are they different?

SIMILARITIES	DIFFERENCES

Based on these two reviews, what have you learned about DNP Projects?

1.
2.
3.

Was there a plan for dissemination? If yes, what was it?

What questions do you still have?

1.
2.
3.

SUMMARY

Viewing completed DNP Projects provides guidance and direction along your DNP Project development. *Scholarly writing is of importance.* It reflects your high level of practice and scholarship, as well as adds to the rigor of your scholarly project. As you read completed DNP Projects, you might observe poor sentence structure, improper punctuation, poor grammar, lack of American Psychological Association (APA) style, and other deficiencies. If you struggle with academic writing, please seek assistance early and often. Get or hire someone to proofread your work. Your ability to communicate in writing reflects on the professionalism of our nursing community. Please give your writing or writing development the attention it deserves.

NEXT STEPS

- Continue to read and review DNP Projects, especially those related to your topic.
- Incorporate faculty feedback.
- Investigate writing support.

REFERENCES AND RESOURCES

American Association of Colleges of Nursing. (2015). *The doctor of nursing practice: Current issues and clarifying recommendations. [White paper].* https://www.aacnnursing.org/Portals/42/News/White-Papers/DNP-Implementation-TF-Report-8-15.pdf

American Association of Colleges of Nursing. (2021). *The essentials: Core competencies for professional nursing education.* https://www.aacnnursing.org/Education-Resources/AACN-Essentials

American Association of Colleges of Nursing. (2023). *Doctor of nursing practice (DNP) tool kit.* https://www.aacnnursing.org/our-initiatives/education-practice/doctor-of-nursing-practice/tool-kit

Dols, J., Hernandez, C., & Miles, H. (2017). The DNP project: Quandaries for nursing scholars. *Nursing Outlook, 65*(1), 84–93. https://doi.org/10.1016/j.outlook.2016.07.009

Rousch, K., & Tesoro, M. (2018). An examination of the rigor and value of the final scholarly projects completed by DNP nursing students. *Journal of Professional Nursing, 34*(6), 437–443. https://doi.org/10.1016/j.profnurs.2018.03.003

Waldrop, J., Carusol, D., Fuchs, M., & Hypes, K. (2014). EC as PIE: Five criteria for executing a successful DNP final project. *Journal of Professional Nursing, 30*(4), 300–306. https://doi.org/10.1016/j.profnurs.2014.01.003

RELATED TEXTBOOK

Bonnel, W., & Smith, K. (2018). *Proposal writing for clinical nursing and DNP projects.* Springer Publishing Company.

LESSON 2.10

THE DNP EXPERIENCE AND PRACTICE HOURS

BACKGROUND

When nurses hear "clinical" or "clinical practice," they commonly envision nursing school and activities related to direct patient care. That experience was necessary to train you as a general nurse and perhaps an advanced practice nurse. But for the most part, the traditional sense of the clinical experience for nurses has to do with preparing you for your role in nursing.

As you recall, the DNP is an advanced degree and not a role in nursing. However, certain skills and competencies informed by the *Essentials* (American Association of Colleges of Nursing [AACN], 2021) are expected of all nurses. The *Essentials* (AACN, 2021) put forth guidance on the expectations for competency as a professional nurse and are divided into Level 1 for entry-level professional nursing education sub-competencies and Level 2 for advanced-level nursing education sub-competencies and specialty/role requirements/competencies. The DNP degree builds upon Level 1 skills and competencies to achieve Level 2 goals. To become an expert on the *Essentials*, you must have a learning experience to ensure that you are prepared at the highest levels of practice. The "DNP practice experience" occurs as part of your DNP academic curriculum and is designed to immerse you in opportunities for both direct and indirect care experiences and is referred to as practicum. The DNP Project is a significant part of this "DNP practice experience." However, some of the *Essentials* may also be learned as part of certain coursework depending on the design of your curriculum. Clearly, the DNP practice experience is not necessarily the same as one may imagine "clinical" in other parts of nursing education. Your DNP practicum experience should directly relate to your professional growth in meeting the *Essentials*.

The AACN (2021) states that to be expert in the *Essentials*, competencies and sub-competencies need to be met. The DNP practice experience should be diverse and not purely focused on direct patient care. Students can be placed in nontraditional environments to expand their knowledge of health-related issues. Faculty members oversee and guide DNP practicum experiences for the student to demonstrate meeting Level 2 sub-competencies and any relevant specialty competencies. Various practicum experiences are possible, as students could be placed with social workers, legislative representatives, attorneys, chief financial officers, pharmaceutical/insurance companies, the military, and other entities involved in healthcare. Be ready to expand activities beyond the nursing profession, as one of the domains is about "interprofessional partnerships." Be clear on how each experience is helping you to advance your competency of the *Essentials* and/or the agenda of the DNP Project.

LEARNING OBJECTIVES

- Review the AACN competencies to address practice experience.
- Discuss practicum expectations for the DNP practice experience at your intended academic institution.

ACTIVITIES

Read the *Essentials* (AACN, 2021, pp. 21–26). Schedule a meeting with your faculty/academic advisor and discuss the following:

- How do you track the completion of your practicum experiences?
- How do you demonstrate meeting competencies through your practicum hours?
- Develop a chart to relate DNP practice activities to the domains of the *Essentials*.
- How is the DNP practice experience executed at your school?
- Who is responsible for "approving" the activities of the DNP practice experience?

SUMMARY

In a subsequent chapter, the DNP practice experience will be explicated further and examples of potential activities presented. Clarify any questions as you begin the DNP Project process. As a sidenote, keeping a log of the DNP project-related activities can be beneficial. A form to assist you with this is provided in the Appendix of the workbook.

NEXT STEPS:

- Review your academic instituion's policy on group DNP Projects before beginning the next activity.

REFERENCES AND RESOURCES

American Association of Colleges of Nursing. (2006). *Doctor of nursing practice essentials*. http://www.nationalacademies.org/hmd/Reports/2010/The-Future-of-Nursing-Leading-Change-Advancing-Health/Report-Brief.aspx

American Association of Colleges of Nursing. (2021). *The essentials: Core competencies for professional nursing education*. https://www.aacnnursing.org/Education-Resources/AACN-Essentials

LESSON 2.11

GROUP DNP PROJECTS

BACKGROUND

According to the American Association of Colleges of Nursing (AACN, 2015), group DNP Projects are acceptable when appropriate to the program and practice area. Like all group projects, it is difficult to determine the exact contributions of each group member without good planning, clear expectations, and a sound process for evaluation. In this lesson, we will examine the pros and cons of group DNP Projects.

Indviduals in favor of group DNP Projects are those who assert that the technique promotes teamwork and collaboration. Faculty might argue in some cases group DNP Projects are necessary because of faculty shortages, lack of collaborative partnerships, clinical/political limitations, to offset the workload for students and faculty, and to develop more accurate experiences of collaborative projects in practice. These are valid points. Wright et al. (2022) in a review of the literature found overarching challenges of DNP Projects consisting of scholarly writing, faculty preparation, and project sustainability. Are these challenges increased by multiple students on a group project? Or could this potentially lessen the burden on faculty and students? These are good questions and necessitate continued conversations.

The AACN (2015) was not against the idea of group DNP Projects given that certain standards are met. Specifically, AACN (2015) informs that "each DNP student must have a leadership role in at least one component of the project and be held accountable for a deliverable" (p. 4). AACN (2015, p. 4) also states that guidelines for the project and a rubric for individual student evaluation must be established at the beginning of the DNP Project process. Examples are provided to support these positions.

LEARNING OBJECTIVES

- Size up the pros and cons of a group DNP Project.
- Decide whether your DNP Project will be an individual or group project.
- Cultivate expectations for planning and evaluation if a group project is selected.

ACTIVITY

Read "The Doctor of Nursing Practice: Current Issues and Clarifying Recommendations, section II on DNP Projects" focusing on group projects on pp. 3–5 (AACN, 2015). https://www.aacnnursing.org/Portals/42/DNP/DNP-Implementation.pdf

Review the requirements for DNP Projects at your academic institution to determine whether a group project is a possibility. If your school does not permit group projects, you can proceed to the chapter summary. If the school does permit group projects, start by reviewing a completed group DNP Project from your school if available. Then answer the questions that follow. When you are finished, we suggest scheduling a meeting with the appropriate faculty member to discuss the group project further. Questions to consider:

- How many students can work in a group?
- How are the groups determined?
- How is each student graded and evaluated as an individual?
- Have group projects been successful in the past?
- Is there a project-planning form the school recommends using to get organized?
- What happens if one of the students is not able to finish the project?
- What happens if one student is completing the work successfully and other members are not?

Faculty should insist on compliance with the AACN (2015, p. 4) recommendations for group projects and agree on the number of students per project in advance. To assist, a planning form to use for group projects is included in the Appendix.

Pros and Cons of Group Projects:

PROS OF GROUP PROJECTS	CONS OF GROUP PROJECTS
Decreases burnout of mentors at project sites as fewer project sites are needed.	Highest terminal degree, fewer and each individual should be evaluated separately.
Provides real experiences and leadership building, as clinical projects are usually collaborative.	If an individual of the group has to have an altered plan of study and leave the project, it is difficult for the other members and may derail the entire project.
	Dissemination plan (e.g., publishing) can cause difficulties if not discussed up front as to who will be first author, and so on.
1.	1.
2.	2.
3.	3.

NEXT STEPS

- If you are going to be doing a group DNP Project, list pros and cons for your project and then complete the planning form.
- Schedule a meeting to discuss your plans with your faculty or academic/project advisor.

REFERENCES AND RESOURCES

American Association of Colleges of Nursing. (2015). *The doctor of nursing practice: Current issues and clarifying recommendations.* https://www.aacnnursing.org/Portals/0/PDFs/Publications/DNP-Implementation.pdf

Forehand, J., Leigh, K., Farrell, R., & Spurlock, A. (2016). Social dynamics in group work. *Teaching and Learning in Nursing, 11*(2), 62–66. https://doi.org/10.1016/j.teln.2015.12.007

Wright, R., Lee, Y., Yoo, A., McIltrot, K., VanGraafeiland, B., Saylor, M., Taylor, J., & Han, H. (2022). *Journal of Professional Nursing, 41*, 53–57.

CHAPTER SUMMARY

Now you have a basic understanding of the DNP degree and DNP Project. We have gone through some of the fundamental information. We compared the terminal nursing degrees of DNP versus PhD. We examined requirements and read completed DNP Projects. Take a moment to reflect on what you have learned:

After completing the lessons, I learned:

I still have questions about:

I am going to take this knowledge and put it into action. Two specific things I need to do are:

1.

2.

3

Identifying Problems and Project Topics

Editor: Molly Bradshaw
Contributors: Tracy R. Vitale, Mercedes Echevarria, Patricia Hindin, Jill Cornelison, Sharon Lock, and Maureen Anderson

Lessons

Lesson 3.1 Your Initial Ideas

Lesson 3.2 Identifying Global and National Problems

Lesson 3.3 Identifying State and Local Problems

Lesson 3.4 Problems With the Healthcare System, Information, and Technology

Lesson 3.5 Cognitive Walkthrough

Lesson 3.6 Networking to Identify and Discuss Problems

Lesson 3.7 Organizing Your Findings

Lesson 3.8 Selecting the Problem and Drafting the Problem Statement

OBJECTIVES

DNP students struggle to identify problems that would make suitable topics for their DNP Projects. In this chapter, the student will complete a series of exercises to help them think through and brainstorm ideas for the project. Students who have already identified a topic will still benefit by completing the lessons to ensure that they have fully examined their ideas. The goal is to identify a problem of interest and draft a problem statement. By the end of this chapter, you will be able to

- Inventory potential DNP Project topics at the global, national, and local levels.
- Examine health-related problems within the context of systems, technology, and policy.
- Explain the impact of health problems on populations.
- Select an appropriate problem as the topic of the DNP Project.
- Draft a problem statement.

INTRODUCTION

In 1953, Alex Faickney Osborn wrote a book titled *Applied Imagination*. In the book, he coined the term *brainstorming*. *Brainstorming* refers to the process of creating ideas and writing them down without critiquing them. We will use guided brainstorming as a way to collect ideas and write them down to inspire the topic of your DNP Project. Later, you will critique them and present the outcome to your faculty.

Ideas for DNP Projects are based on problems. When I ask DNP students about their project topics, I will *always* begin by asking them this question, "What is the *problem* that you have identified?" I follow up by saying next, "How does that impact patients?" It will be helpful for you to adopt this strategy. If you talk about your project, start by stating the problem. Follow up by explaining how it impacts patients or a population. At this point, you should refrain from talking about the intervention of the project. Don't let your mind be distracted or jump ahead in the process. "I am going to educate . . ." or "I am going to do a chart audit . . ."—no, stop! These ideas are premature for now. Keep them written down, but off to the side. The intervention is not informed until you can fully understand what the problem is and what issues impact the problem.

In my experience, post-master's DNP students tend to have an easier time identifying the problem they want to address because they are already working in a nursing role. These students tend to struggle more later in the process when the intervention turns out to be different from what they have envisioned. They take feedback with hesitation and sometimes reluctance, or at least I did. As we move through the lessons in this chapter, I ask that you keep an open mind. Your project problem, intervention, and evaluation plan will evolve as you go through the process. Even if you already have a project topic, problem, or practice gap in mind, you need to complete the work of this chapter to ensure that you have thoroughly brainstormed and considered the problem from every angle.

In contrast, students who are in BSN–DNP programs struggle in a different way. There is enormous pressure because they are completing the DNP degree and training for a new nursing role at the same time. In my experience, these students sometimes feel indifferent to the DNP Project because they are more focused on finishing the requirements for advanced practice or a new nursing role. If BSN–DNP students are asked to identify problems, they will most likely identify problems that they have experienced or observed as an RN. They are also more likely to describe problems at their current place of employment, which often changes after they graduate. Likely, the BSN–DNP student may not be working at all as they go through school and that heightens their anxiety as they hear classmates talking about projects in their place of employment.

I would like to just offer some friendly advice to BSN–DNP students. First, you have to consider what you want your doctoral expertise to be related to. What will advance your career more? Doing a project related to your current role/situation? Doing a project related to the role you are transitioning to? Second, you do not have to be employed by an organization to do a project there. Consider partnering with the organization you want to work for in the future. This same advice might apply to the post-master's DNP student looking to change their career trajectory or organization in the future. It is simply food for thought. Please consult your faculty to discuss this further.

Problems are also experienced in the context of organizations. This brings us to our next point. The topic of your DNP Project will have to be a problem that both you and your stakeholders identify as a priority. Often, problems are broad, and there may be flexibility as it translates to a DNP Project. In other circumstances, an organization may be very specific about the problem they need help with. You will need to have detailed discussions with your faculty and organizational representatives to sort out the exact context of the problem. Eventually, you will need to do more investigation or root-cause analysis once the priority is identified. Your task now is simply to find problems.

Most importantly, problems in the healthcare setting are experienced by patients, families, and populations. We want you to think about the problem from every possible angle. What is the experience of those we serve with this problem? Find inspiration from your population and then consider where this population exists in daily life. Healthcare does not always occur in the four walls of a building, hospital, or clinic.

In summary, remember that these lessons are intended to spark a massive, yet organized brainstorm. Our goal is to ensure that you have fully explored potential problems that could translate to your project topic. In the end, you need to make a final selection and discuss it with your faculty. We will draft a problem statement, and you will be able to revise it in the first lesson of Chapter 4. You may need to revisit this chapter multiple times to reach this goal. Let's begin.

REFERENCE AND RESOURCE

Osborn, A. F. (1953). *Applied imagination*. Scribner's.

MY GOALS FOR IDENTIFYING PROBLEMS AND PROJECT TOPICS ARE TO:

_____
_____
_____
_____
_____
_____
_____
_____
_____
_____
_____
_____
_____
_____
_____
_____

LESSON 3.1

YOUR INITIAL IDEAS

BACKGROUND

Upon admission to DNP programs, students are often asked about a topic for their DNP Project. Some students have well-developed ideas, and this chapter helps enrich those thoughts. Other students are not sure where to start. Start here. Our goal is to help you identify the problem you will work on for your DNP Project. Keep an open mind. Remember that brainstorming is meant for exploring ideas, not critiquing ideas (Stausmire & Ulrich, 2015). The purpose of this lesson is to document initial thoughts, ideas, and experiences as potential topics for the DNP Project. It is the first in a series of brainstorming sessions. The activity is broken down into three parts: your initial thoughts, your favorite clinical subject, and your experiences.

LEARNING OBJECTIVES

- Document, in detail, what you have been thinking about related to the project.
- List your favorite clinical subjects, topics, and diagnosis.
- Reflect on your own experiences.
- Catalog your top three ideas.

ACTIVITIES

This is a brainstorming session. The goal is to document your ideas. Respond to each prompt. Set a timer allowing 5 minutes for each prompt. Write whatever comes to mind—sentences, phrases, or words. Avoid trying to edit, analyze, or get it just right. We will help you with that later. (Editable versions of these activities may be accessed at connect.springerpub.com/content/book/978-0-8261-7484-0/chapter/ch03.)

Brainstorming Prompt 1: Your Initial Thoughts About the DNP Project

When you started the DNP program, what were you considering for your project? Why?

Brainstorming Prompt 2: Your Favorite Clinical Subject

Make a list of your favorite clinical subjects, topics, or diagnoses and explain why you like them.

CLINICAL SUBJECT	WHY I LIKE THIS SUBJECT
Example, Diabetes	Interesting, I have a family history, relevant to family nurse practitioners (FNPs)

Brainstorming Prompt 3: Your Experiences

In your experience (personal or professional), what are the healthcare problems that frustrate you the most? Why? Think of this in terms of patients, families, populations, healthcare organizations/systems, policies, technology, colleagues, and so on.

NEXT STEPS

Now, take a highlighter and review what you have read. Highlight the three ideas that you like the most. Write those ideas next using only two to three words. At the end of the chapter, we will come back to these three concepts.

Example: Distress in diabetics

1. _____
2. _____
3. _____

- Review this article on finding meaningful projects (www.aacn.org/docs/cemedia/C1563.pdf). This article is the first in a series of four articles about starting the quality improvement (QI) process. You may find the content informative.
- Discuss your thoughts with your DNP faculty.

REFERENCE AND RESOURCE

Stausmire, J., & Ulrich, C. (2015). Making it meaningful: Finding quality improvement projects worthy of your time, effort, and expertise. *Critical Care Nurse, 35*(6), 57–62. https://doi.org/10.4037/ccn2015232

LESSON 3.2

IDENTIFYING GLOBAL AND NATIONAL PROBLEMS

BACKGROUND

The first step of the DNP Project is to identify a problem of interest. Problems may have different contexts if they are examined at different levels. For example, the global priorities for vaccine-preventable diseases may be different from national priorities. What if vaccines were readily available in one country but not in another? The problems and issues would be different.

Ultimately, the DNP Project is narrowed to a single focus. The goal here is not to solve the problems of the world. The point is to learn about the potential for global and national priorities to connect or inform your work. Examining global and national health agendas will give you a broad place to start, especially if you have no idea what you want to do your project on. Global issues filter to national issues, which trickle down to state and local issues.

LEARNING OBJECTIVES

- Identify several global and national health priorities.
- List three priorities of interest to you.

ACTIVITIES

The World Health Organization (WHO) is a leader of global health. Visit the WHO website (www.who.int). Review the topics and explore those of interest to you. To look at a more focused list, examine the *Health-related Millennium Development Goals and Targets*. Take notes as you go. Remember, don't try to overanalyze. Go to what draws you in. (Editable versions of these activities may be accessed at connect.springerpub.com/content/book/978-0-8261-7484-0/chapter/ch03.)

Topic:	Notes:
Topic:	Notes:
Topic:	Notes:
Topic:	Notes:
Topic:	Notes:

3 • Identifying Problems and Project Topics   71

☑ **Highlight and list your three favorite global health topics.**

1. _____
2. _____
3. _____

☑ **Visit the Healthy People website (www.healthypeople.gov).**

Review the Healthy People 2020 topics and the proposed Healthy People 2030 topics. Explore those of interest to you. Take notes as you go. Remember, don't try to overanalyze. Go to what draws you in.

Topic:	Notes:
Topic:	Notes:
Topic:	Notes:
Topic:	Notes:
Topic:	Notes:

NEXT STEPS

Highlight and list your favorite three national health topics.

1. _____
2. _____
3. _____

We return to these lists at the end of the chapter. Remember that the global and national health agendas help to articulate needs. Healthcare organizations often set their goals to be in alignment with these. These sites are not comprehensive but are great places to start. To further explore global and national health priorities, see the suggested websites in the section "References and Resources." You can adjust your list as needed.

REFERENCES AND RESOURCES

Centers for Disease Control and Prevention. (2019). *Population health*. https://www.cdc.gov/nccd php/dph/index.html
Centers for Medicare & Medicaid Services. (2019). *Outcome measures*. https://www.cms.gov/Medicare/Quality-Initiatives-Patient-Assessment-Instruments/HospitalQualityInits/OutcomeMeasures.html
U.S. Department of Health and Human Services. (2019). *Healthy people*. https://www.healthypeople.gov
World Health Organization. (2019a). *Health-related millennium development goals and targets*. https://www.who.int/gho/mdg/goals_targets/en
World Health Organization. (2019b). *Topics*. https://www.who.int

> **RELATED TEXTBOOK**
>
> Rosa, W. (2017). *A new era of global health*. Springer Publishing Company.

LESSON 3.3

IDENTIFYING STATE AND LOCAL PROBLEMS

BACKGROUND

This chapter is about brainstorming. We are gathering information to help solidify the idea for your DNP Project. The information being gathered is essentially a list of problems, conditions, and experiences that pique your interest. Later, we will make sense of the information.

In this lesson, we look around at our regional, state, and local environments. What are the pressing health problems? For example, I live in Kentucky. Tobacco abuse and misuse is a major health problem. The problem of tobacco abuse could result in a number of health-related problems such as asthma, chronic obstructive pulmonary disease (COPD), or a health risk factor. Are the local problems cultural? What populations live in your area? Is there a lack of resources? Are there problems with access to care? You are more likely to be aware of issues at this level, but we will still utilize online resources to explore further.

LEARNING OBJECTIVES

- Determine health priorities by visiting websites and writing down what you know.
- List the top three health problems of interest to you.

ACTIVITIES

Start this session by visiting the Centers for Disease Control and Prevention (CDC) website (www.cdc.gov.). In the search bar, select your state and explore the information presented. Also visit your official state agency for health's website. Make a list of health problems of interest to you and take notes as you go. Remember, don't analyze the list yet. Just write down what piques your interest. (Editable versions of these activities may be accessed at connect.springerpub.com/content/book/978-0-8261-7484-0/chapter/ch03.)

State: _____

Topic:	Notes:
Topic:	Notes:
Topic:	Notes:
Topic:	Notes:
Topic:	Notes:

☑ **Highlight and list three keywords from what you have written about a health-related problem.**

1. _____
2. _____
3. _____

☑ **Most likely you are already aware of local health problems. However, make sure that you fully explore the available information. First, see whether you can identify local agencies involved in healthcare. Make a list of the agencies and then, if they have websites, look at the sites. If you can visit the agencies in person, that may also be a great way to network and learn more about local health problems. Second, think about health in your communities—your schools, your place of worship, and your local government. Remember that healthcare does not always occur in a healthcare facility. Finally, talk to people: network. You may discover perspectives that you have not considered.**

Local Agency Name: Health Problems/Priorities:	Notes:
Local Agency Name: Health Problems/Priorities:	Notes:
Local Agency Name: Health Problems/Priorities:	Notes:
Local Agency Name: Health Problems/Priorities:	Notes:
Local Agency Name: Health Problems/Priorities:	Notes:

NEXT STEPS

Circle the three agencies most of interest to you. Make a list of three local health problems of interest to you. At the end of this chapter, we return to this list. If you feel overwhelmed at this point, remember that we will analyze our work later. The goal at this time is to gather information. Analysis of information is discussed later.

1. _____
2. _____
3. _____

RELATED TEXTBOOK

Ervin, N. E., & Kulbok, P. (2018). *Advanced public and community health nursing*. Springer Publishing Company.

LESSON 3.4

PROBLEMS WITH THE HEALTHCARE SYSTEM, INFORMATION, AND TECHNOLOGY

BACKGROUND

When problems in healthcare arise, they are often a result of a faulty system (Institute of Medicine [IOM], 1999). To practice at the highest level, DNP graduates are skilled in identifying problems, making changes, and evaluating the impact of the change. Often, there are problems in the healthcare system that need to be changed. Changes might occur on different system levels.

Information and technology have a close relationship with health systems. Let's first consider information. As information is generated, it can be used to evaluate and improve practice. Information about patients must be communicated and passed from one healthcare team member to another. Patients must be able to access and interpret their health information. Next, consider the impact of technology. Ideally, technology should be a means to improve system issues like scheduling, communication, or access to information. Is that always the case? No, because technology is rarely perfect. It can improve some system issues and cause others.

In this exercise, you can take a few different approaches:

- Examine the system where you are currently employed.
- Examine the system of a place you have worked in the past.
- Examine the system where you hope to be employed in the future.
- Examine a system like your community: a school, place of worship, or club.
- Examine the system as if you were a patient with a given condition.
- Other: _____

You can repeat this exercise in the future if needed. Highlight the option you select so that you can discuss it later with faculty.

LEARNING OBJECTIVES

- Identify the system you are going to examine in this exercise.
- Organize problems and challenges as either macro- or micro-system related.
- State the potential for impact by information.
- State the potential for impact by technology.

ACTIVITIES

Systems thinking provides a good framework to begin problem identification (Figure 3.1). Write down potential problems for each level.

Patient Level

Problem of Interest: _____

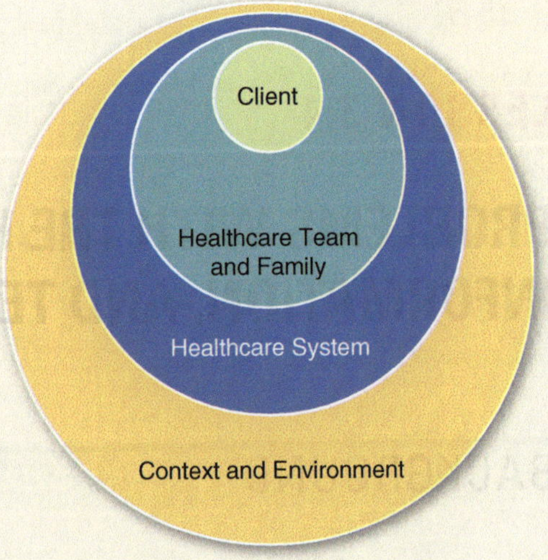

76 The DNP Project Workbook

Care-Team Level

Problem of Interest: _____
_____

Organizational Level

Problem of Interest: _____
_____

Environmental Level

Problem of Interest: _____

Figure 3.1 The levels of systems thinking.

☑ **Consider the potential impact of information. Write a statement about the impact of information on the system problems.**
_____

☑ **Consider the potential impact of technology. Write a statement about the impact of technology on the system problems.**
_____

Review your work on this activity to date. Highlight and list three key problems. List them here:

1. _____
2. _____
3. _____

If you are following the workbook lessons in order, we are starting to gather several problems. You may or may not notice overlap. Remember, do not try to analyze anything yet. We are working toward a summary and synthesis. For now, continue to gather ideas and deepen your understanding of various problems. In a later chapter, we talk more about organizational assessment and workflow analysis. You are doing great! Keep going. Work hard.

NEXT STEPS

- Talk to your DNP faculty.
- Continue to be alert for opportunities to improve systems and technology use.

REFERENCES AND RESOURCES

Bisht, C., Mehrotra, D., & Kalra, P. (2019). *To calculate the usability of healthcare mobile applications using cognitive walkthrough*. https://link.springer.com/chapter/10.1007/978-981-13-1642-5_24

Institute of Medicine. (1999). *To err is human*. National Academies Press.

The Office of the National Coordinator for Health Information Technology. (2019). *Topics*. https://www.healthit.gov/topics

Sheehan, B., & Bakken, S. (n.d.). *Approaches to workflow analysis in healthcare settings*. https://www.ncbi.nlm.nih.gov/pmc/articles/PMC3799136/pdf/amia_2012_ni_371.pdf

Stalter, A. M., Phillips, J. M., Ruggiero, J. S., Scardaville, D. L., Merriam, D., Dolansky, M. A., Goldschmidt, K. A., Wiggs, C. M., & Winegardner, S. (2017). A concept analysis of systems thinking. *Nursing Forum*, *52*(4), 323–330. https://doi.org/10.1111/nuf.12196

RELATED TEXTBOOK

McBride, S., & Tietze, M. (2018). *Nursing informatics for the advanced practice nurse: Patient safety, quality, outcomes, and interprofessionalism* (2nd ed.). Springer Publishing Company.

Chapter 9: Workflow Redesign

LESSON 3.5

COGNITIVE WALKTHROUGH

BACKGROUND

Cognitive walkthrough is a technique used to evaluate process and determine ease of usability. It helps to identify problems. DNP students may or may not have access to the site where their DNP Projects will take place in the beginning of the planning process. If you do have access, you may find it more helpful to do a live, literal walkthrough of the workspace in this exercise. If you do not have access, just use experience, imagination, and critical thinking skills to do a "cognitive" walkthrough.

LEARNING OBJECTIVES

- Document potential problems in the context of your setting.

ACTIVITIES

In this lesson, you will be guided through a series of prompts. As you complete the lesson, your goal is to focus on the perspective of the patient.

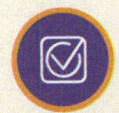

✓ Describe the patient.

- Do they have a certain condition?
- Does the patient have any impairment?
- What does this patient need to improve their health?

✓ Imagine that the patient has entered the health system.

- In what context: community, outpatient, or inpatient?
- How does the patient find access?
- What is it like when the patient arrives?

✓ Walk through the environment and the interactions the patient will have with staff.

- Have you identified any problems?

✓ Now imagine the patient's care is in transition.

- In what context: community, outpatient, or inpatient?
- What types of communications need to take place?
- Does the patient have the resources they need?
- Have you identified any problems?

SUMMARY

In later chapters, we talk more about formal organizational assessment and process mapping. The point here is to critically think about what problems a patient might encounter. It is an informal strategy to get you thinking about potential problems. You will organize your chapter findings in the next activity.

LESSON 3.6

NETWORKING TO IDENTIFY AND DISCUSS PROBLEMS

BACKGROUND

Networking with others adds perspective. Just because you identify that something is a problem, it does not mean that others perceive it in the same way. Networking also creates connections that may lead to collaboration in the future. In this lesson, it may be helpful for you to utilize some of the tips we suggested in the beginning of the workbook. As you network, be sure to leave your business card with people. Organize information from the discussions by taking notes that include the time and date. Later, you may want to incorporate the discussion in your DNP Project proposal. The conversation can be recorded as a "personal communication."

Whom should I network with? To begin, we recommend starting with your faculty. Review the faculty profiles at your school. If possible, schedule a meeting with faculty who have expertise in your area of interest. Then, you may consider networking with a stakeholder in one or two of the organizations/systems you identified. Who are the leaders there whom you will need to know to make change?

We also recommend networking with others in your current or future nursing role. If you are a nurse executive, talk to other nurse executives. If you are a BSN–DNP student transitioning to a role as a pediatric nurse practitioner, talk to other pediatric nurse practitioners. Professional organizations often have outlets for connecting to online discussion forums. You can also join the Doctor of Nursing Practice Organization for free (www.doctorsofnursingpractice.org). This organization is the only national organization for DNP-prepared nurses, but it is not specific to the nursing role.

LEARNING OBJECTIVES

- Engage in networking.
- Discuss problems of interest to colleagues, stakeholders, and others.

ACTIVITIES

Use this outline to begin your networking journey. For the purposes of finding the problem you want to work on for your project, we recommend that you network with at least three people. Review the suggested questions, which are all open ended to begin conversation. As you interact, you can ask more pointed questions. Remember to get contact information so that you can reach out again in the future. Be on time, be gracious, and thank people for their input. (Editable versions of these activities may be accessed at connect.springerpub.com/content/book/978-0-8261-7484-0/chapter/ch03.)

Start: I am a DNP student at _____. I am interested in _____.

- What have you observed related to _____
  _____

- How does the system, information, technology, or policy impact _____
  _____

- What has been done so far to address _____
  _____
- Are there any discussions on improving _____
  _____
- What are some problems you experienced _____
  _____
- How are problems analyzed _____
  _____

Networking Activity 1

Name:
Organization:

Notes:

Networking Activity 2

Name:
Organization:

Notes:

Networking Activity 3

Name:
Organization:

Notes:

Expert Commentary: Jill Cornelison, DNP, RN

As a faculty advisor for DNP students, I am astutely aware that identification of a clinical problem for a potential DNP Project is not a simple task for the student. Often, students choose a problem they feel passionate about or have become aware of through reading the healthcare literature. Conversely, I encounter students who have already decided what they want to implement for their project or what practice change they want to make without knowing whether a problem actually exists. Difficulties also arise when the clinical problem that the student has chosen does not align with an agency's needs and objectives or the clinical problem does not evolve into the implementation of a scholarly project.

Identifying a clinical problem requires early discussion and analysis of a potential agency's needs. The student should have conversations with leaders within the agency before making a final decision on a clinical problem for the DNP Project. In other words, they need to network. The effort spent on the front end to identify a viable, appropriate, and feasible clinical problem affords the student more opportunity to develop a scholarly DNP Project that impacts healthcare outcomes. Networking is purposeful. It is actively seeking and engaging others who may have common concerns, interests, and goals. You need to get out and put yourself out there. Take advantage of every opportunity to network.

NEXT STEPS

- Network to align your goals with the needs of the organization/agency.
- Determine the timelines for your project and the agency's need.

RELATED TEXTBOOK

Marshall, E. S., & Broome, M. E. (2016). *Transformational leadership in nursing.* Springer Publishing Company.
  Chapter 5: Collaborative Leadership Contexts: Networks, Communication, Decision-Making, and Motivation

NOTES

LESSON 3.7

ORGANIZING YOUR FINDINGS

BACKGROUND

As discussed earlier, brainstorming is a process of generating ideas without judgment. Problems are the foundation of DNP Projects. You have been completing a series of exercises to identify problems. Now we begin the process of organizing the information. After it is consolidated, we will begin critiquing the information and move toward selecting the problem for your DNP Project.

LEARNING OBJECTIVES

- List the top findings from each activity in its designated location.
- Analyze the information and select your two favorite problems.

ACTIVITIES

Reflection

Write a short summary of your new perspective of health-related problems after completing the previous activities.

Transfer your lists from previous activities completed in this chapter to their designated locations here. Then, take some time to reflect on the content. After careful reflection, highlight the top two problems of interest to you and write them down. (Editable versions of these activities may be accessed at connect.springerpub.com/content/book/978-0-8261-7484-0/chapter/ch03.)

3 • Identifying Problems and Project Topics   **83**

ORGANIZING YOUR FINDINGS:
Problems I Have Identified
Transfer your lists from each
lesson to this page.

Initial Ideas:
Initial Thoughts, Subjects, and Experiences

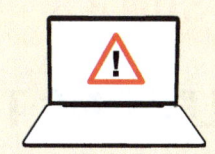

1.
2.
3.

Problems with Systems, Information, and Technology:

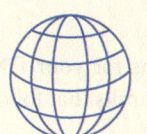

1.
2.
3.

Global Problems:

1.
2.
3.

National Problems:

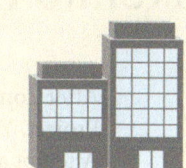

1.
2.
3.

State and Local Problems:

1.
2.
3.

fter Networking, These **Problems Were Identified:**

1.
2.
3.

Selection

1. Highlight similar problems in the same color.
2. Highlight your *favorite* problem.
3. Circle your top two choices and list them here.

Selected Problem A: _____

Selected Problem B: _____

Are you pleased with these topics?

Notes:

Write your selected problems here.

PROBLEM A:

PROBLEM B:

NEXT STEPS

- Discuss your top two ideas with your faculty.

LESSON 3.8

SELECTING THE PROBLEM AND DRAFTING THE PROBLEM STATEMENT

BACKGROUND

After completing the brainstorming process, you have identified two potential problems for your DNP Project. You must discuss them with your faculty or DNP Project chair. Complete the prompts that follow. Attempt a draft of your DNP Project problem statement.

LEARNING OBJECTIVES

- Discuss with your faculty the potential problems you have identified.
- Finalize your choice for the problem of interest in your DNP Project.
- Draft a problem statement.

ACTIVITIES

In this activity, you will do a side-by-side comparison of the two problems you identified in the previous lesson. After listing each problem, complete the prompts to share with your DNP faculty. This may also provide perspective if you are "torn" between two project ideas. (Editable versions of these activities may be accessed at connect.springerpub.com/content/book/978-0-8261-7484-0/chapter/ch03.)

PROBLEM A:

_____

I selected this problem because:

_____

_____

_____

_____

PROBLEM B:

_____

I selected this problem because:

_____

_____

_____

_____

I know it's a problem because: I know it's a problem because:

_____   _____

_____   _____

_____   _____

_____   _____

Tips From Faculty Experts

Finding the Middle Ground for the Student and Clinical Agency

Sharon Lock, PhD, APRN, FNAP, FAANP

Many students enter a DNP program without an idea about what they want to do their project on. They know they have to do a project but haven't put much thought into it. During initial discussions, I try to find out, in general, what topics students are interested in. If a clinical agency has a need for a quality improvement (QI) study that a student could be a part of, that could be a win-win for both the agency and the student. However, the time frames of the clinical agency and the student may not coincide. Typically, the time frame for DNP Projects is over a period of years, whereas a clinical agency will want a QI project to be completed in a much shorter time frame.

Often, the student's original idea is broad, and they need help narrowing down the project. I ask students to think about part of the problem that could be managed in a better way. Once the student has narrowed down the topic, I advise the student to go to the literature to see what has been published on the topic. Sometimes, the student finds a study or project that is very similar to what they were interested in doing and gets discouraged. When that happens, we brainstorm about ways to replicate or improve the project. How can it be translated into the context of the clinical agency the student is working at? The key is to find the middle ground—the project that a student can complete for an agency over a period of time that is reasonable for both.

Collaborate With an Open Mind

Maureen Anderson, DNP, APN, CRNA

Identifying a project topic takes an open mind and multiple levels of collaboration. A single idea has the ability to grow into a topic that can have a substantial impact on professional practice. As students start to navigate the DNP process and develop ideas, it is crucial to have conversations with experts in the area of interest. It is through these early conversations that a project truly evolves and takes on a life of its own. These conversations should begin with fellow classmates who share the same novice vantage point and then continue with expert faculty who can focus, validate, and vet an idea. Pairing a novice DNP student with an expert faculty member and clinician lends itself to fresh innovative ideas due to the difference in perspectives and level of experience.

As the project idea is being established and vetted, the conversations can and should continue with stakeholders at a local, state, and even national level. Examples include local private practice groups or state and national professional associations. Making these connections early in the process can set the stage for a DNP Project and create additional opportunities for reporting and dissemination. A project's success can be directly related to the level of collaboration, networking, and a student's open mind.

Problem Before Innovation

Patricia Hindin, PhD, CNM, RYT 200

The initial critical misstep that students often make is that after identifying a topic, they begin formulating their innovation. The proposed change is usually a teaching project with a pre- and posttest questionnaire. So I inquire. What do you really know about the most current literature? And why do you think that people have to be educated about it? What is the problem at your clinical site? You need to analyze the topic and focus the issue and find out what has been done in the literature to address the problem. How successful has the site been with the problem? Why? Why not? Your role as a DNP is to take evidence from the literature and translate that to your specific problem situation.

> **Warning and Critical Point:** Before you begin the selection process, you must have a conversation with your faculty. We recommend against moving forward with the workbook unless you have assurance from your faculty that the problem is viable. Remind the faculty that our goal is to find problems. We have not performed official workflow analysis or explored the potential solutions yet. Bring your work from this chapter with you. Talk about the pros and cons of each problem and utilize this worksheet to help you.

PROBLEM A:

PROBLEM B:

PROS	CONS	PROS	CONS

After discussions with faculty and weighing pros and cons, my final selected problem for my DNP Project is:

_____
_____
_____
_____
_____

The problem statement addresses the practice problem and provides continued direction throughout the duration of the project. It answers the questions of who, what, where, when, why, and how. A problem statement specific to a DNP Project offers the reader an understanding of the issues surrounding the practice problem and the reason the project was selected.

ACTIVITIES

A template statement is provided. Use it to write your own problem statement.

Suggested template for problem statements.

___(Problem)____ is an issue for _(Population)__ because _(provide supporting rationale, evidence, data)__. An opportunity exists to improve outcomes by __(describe proposed intervention)__. The purpose of this DNP Project will be to _(your intended outcome)___.

Example 1

Screening for hepatitis C consistently in the primary care setting is lacking. Providers and their team lack a consistent process. Failure to promptly identify those at risk or with hepatitis C may delay care and result in poor patient outcomes. An opportunity exists to create an evidence-based template in the electronic health records that could improve the screening process and thereby improve rates of referral and treatment. The purpose of this DNP Project will be to develop, implement, and evaluate a new process for hepatitis C screening in the partnering agency.

Example 2

Caregivers often experience negative psychological, behavioral, and physiological effects on their daily lives and health. Many studies have documented the value of conducting interventions to decrease stress for those at risk for developing chronic stress due to being a caregiver. A needs assessment conducted within a parish setting has documented the need to implement these evidence-based interventions to reduce stress outcomes scores and to increase self-rated health in this population. Participation in this stress-reduction program could improve outcomes in African American women experiencing caregiver stress. The purpose of this project will be to implement and evaluate a care delivery model of stress reduction in the parish setting to assist in improving outcomes related to caregiver stress.

Example 3

The COVID-19 pandemic raised awareness regarding the need to improve mental health for nurses. The nursing staff at the partnering agency have identified that they need additional support to relieve stressors experienced during their shift. The administrative team has allocated funding to further develop evidence-based interventions aimed at reducing stress on shift. The purpose of this DNP Project will be to identify, implement, and evaluate one evidence-based strategy for stress reduction.

Example 4

In the partnering oncology clinic, staff have identified a need to improve medication compliance for patients receiving oral chemotherapy. These may not receive the same opportunity for patient education or management of side effects compared to those getting intravenous therapies, which puts them at risk according to both the literature and internal data. A practice change is necessary. Using a bundled, interdisciplinary approach, the nurses and clinical pharmacist will implement a new process for both education and medication monitoring. Ultimately, the goal is to improve medication compliance in this population.

You will notice that these problem statements are not specific as to the details of the project design, project intervention, and project outcomes. The formal review of literature will further guide the project. The goal of the problem statement is to clearly communicate:

- Who is affected?
- What is the problem they are experiencing?
- What proof exists that it is a problem?
- What is the proposed intervention or opportunity to improve?
- What is the primary outcome you want to see? (measurable outcome)

Write your problem statement next to the template:

___(Problem)___ is an issue for _(Population)__ because _(provide supporting rationale, evidence, data)__. An opportunity exists to improve outcomes by __(describe proposed intervention)__. The purpose of this DNP Project will be to _(your intended outcome)___.	

NEXT STEPS

- Take time to reflect on your problem statement.
- Revise the statement as necessary and with the input of your DNP team.
- Remember that this is only a first draft. You will continue to revise the problem statement as you go further in the process.

REFERENCE AND RESOURCE

Hernon, P., & Schwartz, C. (2007). What is a problem statement? *Library & Information Science Research, 29*(3), 307–309. http://www.lis-editors.org/bm~doc/editorial-problem-statement.pdf

> **RELATED TEXTBOOK**
>
> Bonnel, W., & Smith, K. (2018). *Proposal writing for clinical nursing and DNP projects*. Springer Publishing Company.
> Chapter 3: Writing a Good Problem Statement and Putting the Problem in Context

CHAPTER SUMMARY

The focus of this chapter is to identify problems that could potentially translate into the topic of your DNP Project. Problems are broad. Identifying the problem gives you a starting point from which to further develop your project. It is to be hoped that the experience of working on a DNP Project related to this topic will advance your knowledge and skills toward your long-term goals. Solidifying the problem statement adds clarity to your DNP Project.

Reflections

What are two things that you have learned in this chapter?

1.

2.

If you were able to choose a problem for your project, what is your final selection? Why is working on this problem important to you?

_____

_____

_____

_____

_____

If you were not able to select a problem to pursue, we recommend the following actions:

- Can you identify a reason why you are struggling?
- Consult with your faculty.
- Review the lessons and repeat activities as necessary.
- Examine the suggested list of problems in the Appendix.

You should have a problem identified before moving on. Realize that if the problem changes, you may need to repeat these lessons. Additional copies of the forms are located in the online resources of this textbook. If this is the case, do not be discouraged. This is a real-world project subjected to real-world circumstances. The only thing that you can count on is that things change and evolve. Continue to work the process.

NOTES

4

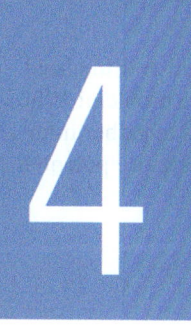

Developing the DNP Project Background and Context

Editor: Molly Bradshaw
Contributors: Tracy R. Vitale and Karen Gilbert

Lessons

Lesson 4.1 Initial Inquiry and Initial Search

Lesson 4.2 Finding Evidence and Data to Document the Problem

Lesson 4.3 Strategic Agendas Related to the Problem

Lesson 4.4 Clinical Guidelines Related to the Problem

Lesson 4.5 Policies Related to the Problem

Lesson 4.6 Using the Quadruple Aim to Examine the Problem

Lesson 4.7 Impact of the Problem on Patients, Families, and Communities: Social Determinants of Health

Lesson 4.8 Impact of the Problem on Organizations

Lesson 4.9 Demonstrating the Value of the DNP Project

Lesson 4.10 Putting It All Together—The DNP Project Outline: Draft #1

OBJECTIVES

After selecting a problem to address for the DNP Project, a problem statement is written and finalized. The next step is to fully describe the background and context of the problem. What is the problem? Who is affected by it? Why is it a problem? In this chapter, students are guided through lessons to gather information about the problem in its local context. After a thorough investigation, students explore potential solutions to address the problem. By the end of this chapter, you will be able to

- Refine the problem statement and describe what is currently known.
- Present the key points of policy, standards, and guidelines related to the problem.
- Examine the problem in its local context.
- List potential solutions to the problem.
- Organize findings in preparation for proposal writing.

INTRODUCTION

The DNP Project is centered on a problem. The problem of interest is both the starting point and the focal point. Starting today, if someone asks you this question, "What is your DNP Project about?" your reply should be, "The problem I am focused on is _____." In this chapter, our goal is to gather information to ensure that you fully understand this problem in its local context. We will help you organize this information so that you are prepared to begin writing the first draft of your project proposal. Our goals for this chapter are to determine

- What is the problem?
- Who is affected by the problem?
- Why is it a problem?

What questions do you have about your problem of interest? For some DNP students, the problem may be a topic with which you have a strong working knowledge and experience. Maybe there is more to learn. A spirit of inquiry will sharpen and broaden your perspective. There may be factors you have overlooked or were not aware of that influence the problem. For other DNP students, the problem may be new. For example, if you are a BSN–DNP student and your faculty is suggesting a problem to you for investigation, you may be starting with a more novice perspective. In either case, we are here to help you discover information and organize the findings to deepen your understanding.

The DNP graduate should be an expert in their project subject matter. At the doctoral level, this is very important. Remember that the American Association of Colleges of Nursing (AACN, 2015) suggests that this is a foundation of future scholarship. Is addressing this problem something that could advance your career, role, or future endeavors? Does addressing the problem add value to the community, organization, or healthcare system? Most importantly, will addressing this problem improve health outcomes for patients, families, and populations?

The lessons and activities in this chapter are the next logical steps of the DNP Project process.

- You are prepared for success.
- You are positioned for leadership.
- You have identified your problem of interest.
- You are moving toward comprehensive investigation of the problem in this chapter.

At the end of the chapter, we guide you toward resources to help you with the writing process. We recommend that you complete all of the lessons in this chapter *before* you begin formal writing. Think of this

REFERENCE AND RESOURCE

American Association of Colleges of Nursing. (2015). *The doctor of nursing practice: Current issues and clarifying recommendations.* https://www.aacnnursing.org/Portals/42/News/White-Papers/DNP-Implementation-TF-Report-8-15.pdf

LESSON 4.1

INITIAL INQUIRY AND INITIAL SEARCH

BACKGROUND

Nurses prepared with the DNP degree are committed to the use of evidence to guide and change when necessary (Christenbery, 2018). When problems are identified, change begins by asking questions. What is the problem? What impacts or influences the problem? The spirit of inquiry drives exploration of data, relationships, phenomena, and practice to better understand the problem's context.

In this lesson, we guide you through the initial inquiries that are necessary for the background of the project. You will need to complete some initial literature searches. The goal at this time is to gather information about the problem. We ask you to track your searches and keep a working reference list.

As the project develops, you will have additional questions that need clarification. What is the best method for _____? What strategies promote adoption of a clinical guideline? To answer these pointed, focused questions, a formal review of the literature, an integrative review, or a systematic review is completed. We discuss the differences in a later lesson. Ultimately, the DNP Project is guided by question(s) you ask (Christenbery, 2018) and the evidence you translate and implement to solve your problem of interest (Holly, 2019).

It is critical to mention the importance of working with librarians. Librarians are trained specifically to help identify and retrieve information. They know the nuances of keywords, Boolean phrasing, and databases. We *highly* recommend that you reach out to your university library and seek assistance *early*. Librarians are invaluable colleagues.

LEARNING OBJECTIVES

- Complete initial searches related to the problem.
- Compile a working reference list with a minimum of 10 references.

94 The DNP Project Workbook

ACTIVITIES

(Editable versions of these activities may be accessed at connect.springerpub.com/content/book/978-0-8261-7484-0/chapter/ch04.)

☑ **Ground Zero.** Ask yourself whether you are informed on your topic. In other words, do you routinely read and consume information on this topic? To become an expert, you need to begin by improving your general knowledge. Make a plan:

1. I will read two to three articles daily starting on: _____ (date).
2. I will explore podcasts on this topic starting on: _____ (date).
3. I will consume information daily on this topic starting on: _____ (date).

☑ **Search the literature on your own using the Internet.** Gather as much information related to your problem as possible. Use this table to help you organize your findings.

Source Citation:	Notes:
1	
2	
3	
4	
5	
6	
7	
8	
9	
10	

Write a short summary of what you have discovered about your problem. Why is it a problem?

Now let's focus on your database searches. Develop a series of keywords based on your problem and population.

SUMMARIZE YOUR PROBLEM IN ONE SENTENCE	SELECT THREE KEYWORDS RELEVANT TO THE PROBLEM
	1. _____ 2. _____ 3. _____

My population of interest is: _____.

Boolean logic is a symbolic method of combining keywords to focus searches (Digital Literacy, 2010; Kate the Librarian, 2011). Here, we focus on the use of "OR." When you type the keywords in a search box with OR (in all caps) between the key terms, the database will produce results with _(Key Term)_ OR _(Key Term)_ (Figure 4.1). The OR operator can be effective when there are terms that are synonymous (or nearly synonymous) to your keywords, saving a second search. For example, kidney disease OR renal disease. The next approach is to use AND (in all caps) between key terms. This will cause the database to combine results that contain both key terms (Figure 4.2).

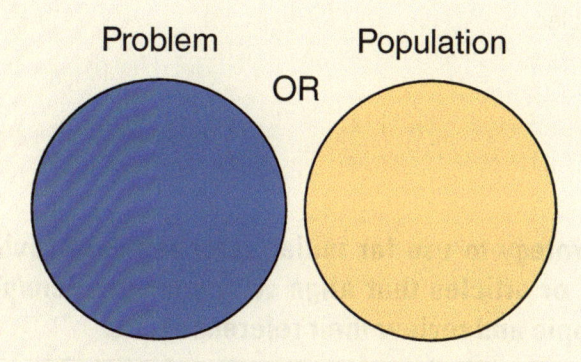

Figure 4.1 Boolean logic: The use of "OR."

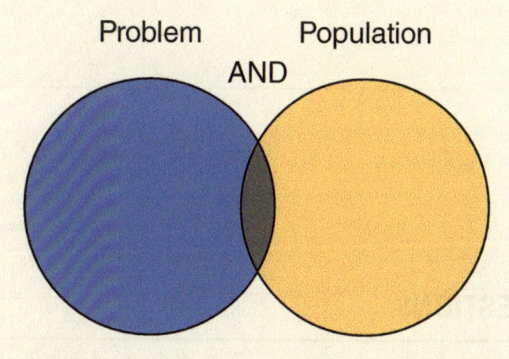

Figure 4.2 Boolean logic: The use of "AND."

☑ **Attempt this search in three to four databases. Document the number of results you get with each search. Review the titles and begin to review information you feel is relevant. Are you finding different information compared to your first searches?**

DATABASE	SEARCH COMBINATION	# OF RESULTS	# OF ITEMS REVIEWED
For example, CINAHL	COPD OR elderly/ COPD AND elderly	110	27
		658	256

CINAHL, Cumulative Index to Nursing and Allied Health Literature; COPD, chronic obstructive pulmonary disease.

Suggested Databases:

- CINAHL
- PubMed
- PsycINFO
- Google Scholar
- Other:

☑ **Another great strategy to use for initial searches is to review the reference lists of completed DNP Projects or articles that align with your problem/population. Find two DNP Projects related to your topic and review their reference lists.**

Project #1: Title _____

Key References:

Project #2: Title _____

Key References:

☑ **ADDITIONAL SUGGESTIONS**

Is there a key journal that deals with your problem? Search this journal.

Is there an author who writes frequently about your problem? Search the author's work.

SUMMARY

The initial inquiry and searches are meant to improve your knowledge and discover basic information about your problem. A tip for students: As a faculty member, I personally want to see the reference list, formatted using the seventh edition of the American Psychological Association (2020) style manual, that a student has complied for an initial search. I generally recommend that it contain 10 references at a minimum, often more. Students will often say, "I have reviewed the literature and. . . ." I stop them immediately. I want to see the reference list. *Exactly*, what have you found so far? It helps me guide students in a more precise way. Next steps:

- Work toward goals set to routinely consume information about your problem.
- Keep a record of your searches and findings to present to faculty.

REFERENCES AND RESOURCES

American Psychological Association. (2020). *Publication manual of the American Psychological Association* (7th ed.). Author.
Christenbery, T. (Ed.). (2018). *Evidence-based practice in nursing*. Springer Publishing Company.
Digital Literacy [Screen name]. (2010, May 14). *Boolean logic* [Video file] https://youtu.be/YlghuxGjHok
Holly, C. (2019). *Practice-based scholarly inquiry and the DNP capstone*. Springer Publishing Company.
Kate the Librarian [Screen name]. (2011, July 11). *Boolean searching basics. [Video file]*. https://youtu.be/jMV7X3W_beg&feature=youtu.be
Sliante Department of Health. (2013). *How to conduct a literature search*. https://health.gov.ie/wp-content/uploads/2015/01/conducting_a_literature_search_2013.pdf

RELATED TEXTBOOKS

Christenbery, T. (Ed.). (2018). *Evidence-based practice in nursing*. Springer Publishing Company.
   Chapter 5: Using Nursing Phenomena to Explore Evidence
   Chapter 6: Evidence-Based Practice: Success of Practice Change Depends on the Question
Holly, C. (2019). *Practice-based scholarly inquiry and the DNP capstone*. Springer Publishing Company.
   Chapter 2: Practice-Based Scholarly Inquiry

LESSON 4.2

FINDING EVIDENCE AND DATA TO DOCUMENT THE PROBLEM

BACKGROUND

To solve a problem, you need proof that the problem exists. You need evidence and data to document the problem and plan for intervention and evaluation. This exercise helps you begin to gather evidence and data. Hickey and Brosnan (2017) outline common sources of evidence used by Doctors of Nursing Practice (DNPs):

- Print and electronic resources (including databases)
- Guidelines and protocols
- Standards for practice
- Observations
- Interviews
- Surveys
- Comparisons
- Personal experiences
- Reflections

You will need to discuss this lesson with your faculty. Determine the policies at your school on interviews, focus groups, needs assessments, and surveys *prior* to conducting them. Ensure that you are compliant with the institutional review board (IRB).

Having data about a problem is compelling. Our world is exploding with data. Electronic health records, personal health records, mobile technology, wearable devices, and public health data are just a few of the data sources that might provide context to your problem. Explore the potential data sources for your problem of interest.

LEARNING OBJECTIVES

- Gather evidence and data to inform the problem of interest.

ACTIVITIES

In this lesson, we are building on the information you found in Lesson 4.2. Some information may be redundant, but that may indicate its importance. We try to use multiple lenses in approaching these activities. Using this table, gather data, information, and evidence related to your problem of interest. Document the source and key points from each. Remember to bookmark them for later reference in writing the DNP Project proposal. Setting this up electronically may be most helpful.

TYPE OF EVIDENCE	SOURCE	KEY POINTS
Print/electronic		
Guidelines/protocols		
Standards of practice		
Observations		
Interviews		
Surveys		

Data

As you partner with an organization to plan for your DNP Project, ask about what data and information the organization has collected to document a problem. The agency may be willing to partner with you to collect information. Ask about its systems for collecting information on process improvement and quality. This will be important later as you plan for your intervention and evaluation of process/outcomes. Identify potential data sources and explore them.

NEXT STEPS

- Continue to explore and collect evidence and data to document your problem.
- Ensure that you explore public databases.

REFERENCES AND RESOURCES

Community Action Toolbox. (n.d.). *Collecting information about a problem.* https://ctb.ku.edu/en/table-of-contents/assessment/assessing-community-needs-and-resources/collect-information/main

Hickey, J. V., & Brosnan, C. A. (Eds.). (2017). *Evaluation of health care quality for DNPs* (2nd ed.). Springer Publishing Company.

RELATED TEXTBOOKS

Hickey, J. V., & Brosnan, C. A. (Eds.). (2017). *Evaluation of health care quality for DNPs* (2nd ed.). Springer Publishing Company.
- Chapter 2: The Nature of Evidence as a Basis for Evaluation
- Chapter 10: Evaluation of Patient Care Based on Standards, Guidelines, and Protocol
- Chapter 11: Healthcare Teams

McBride, S., & Tietze, M. (2019). *Nursing informatics for the advanced practice nurse.* Springer Publishing Company.

Chapter 10: Evaluation Methods for Electronic Health Records
Chapter 11: Electronic Health Records and Health Information Exchanges Providing Value and Results for Patients, Providers, and Healthcare Systems
Chapter 13: Public Health Data to Support Healthy Communities in Health Assessment Planning
Chapter 18: Data Management and Data Analytics: The Foundations for Improvement
Chapter 27: Big Data and Advanced Analytics

LESSON 4.3

STRATEGIC AGENDAS RELATED TO THE PROBLEM

BACKGROUND

A strategic agenda is a set of goals or principles that guide the activity of an organization. For example, Healthy People is a strategic agenda that drives healthcare in the United States. An organization might have goals that help it achieve its mission statement. A healthcare team might develop a strategic plan for a patient, family, or population. In this lesson, you investigate strategic agendas that are related to your problem of interest.

LEARNING OBJECTIVES

- Locate related strategic agendas.
- Explain how they relate to your problem of interest.

ACTIVITIES

Recall our discussion of the Institute of Medicine (IOM) reports *To Err Is Human* (1999), *Crossing the Quality Chasm* (2001), *The Future of Nursing* (2011), and Healthy People. From the perspective of your problem and population of interest, write down the relationships.

STRATEGIC AGENDA	RELATIONSHIP TO YOUR PROBLEM/POPULATION OF INTEREST
Future of Nursing Report	
Healthy People	

STRATEGIC AGENDA	RELATIONSHIP TO YOUR PROBLEM/POPULATION OF INTEREST
Other IOM report:	
Other:	

☑ **At the organizational level, are there strategic agendas that relate to your problem? If so, describe.**

_____
_____

☑ **From the perspective of the healthcare team, are there strategic agendas for patients or populations that are related to your problem? If so, describe.**

_____
_____

NEXT STEPS

- Be alert to strategic agendas at all levels that are related to your problem/populations of interest.
- Continue to build on your findings.

REFERENCES AND RESOURCES

Institute of Medicine. (1999). *To err is human: Building a safer healthcare system*. National Academies Press.
Institute of Medicine. (2001). *Crossing the quality chasm*. National Academies Press.
Institute of Medicine. (2011). *The future of nursing: Leading change, advancing health*. National Academies Press.

RELATED TEXTBOOK

Hickey, J. V., & Brosnan, C. A. (Eds.). (2017). *Evaluation of health care quality for DNPs* (2nd ed.). Springer Publishing Company.
   Chapter 3: Conceptual Models for Evaluation in Advanced Nursing Practice

LESSON 4.4

CLINICAL GUIDELINES RELATED TO THE PROBLEM

BACKGROUND

The DNP degree is practice-focused (American Association of Colleges of Nursing [AACN], 2015). Variation in clinical practice creates potential for risk and ultimate harm to the patient. To streamline practice, utilize evidence, and promote patient safety, use of clinical practice guidelines (CPGs) makes logical sense (Christenbery, 2018). If the CPG is well-developed, it can be used as a cornerstone, guide, and benchmark for the DNP Project.

CPGs are usually developed by an organization to streamline practice and reduce potential harm (Institute of Medicine [IOM], 2011). To best utilize them in a DNP Project, it will be necessary to identify a guideline, understand its context, and formally appraise the content. The IOM (2011) published a document to assist health professionals in determining the quality of guidelines called *Clinical Practice Guidelines We Can Trust*. We use those standards to frame the work of this activity. Nurses may also be in contact with variations of CPGs—protocols, clinical pathways, and care plans—in their work settings. In the book by Christenbery, Table 9.3, Clinical Practice Guideline Terms, outlines and clarifies the differences among guidelines.

LEARNING OBJECTIVES

- Identify a CPG related to your problem of interest.
- Appraise the guideline using the IOM standards.

ACTIVITIES

Use this worksheet to appraise the guideline you have identified. For more details on each standard, refer to the IOM document (http://data.care-statement.org/wp-content/uploads/2016/12/IOMGuidelines-2013-1.pdf).

Problem: _____

Official Title of Selected Guideline: _____

Developer/Source: _____

IOM STANDARD	IS THE STANDARD MET?
Established Transparency: Is the process used to develop the guideline identified?	Yes/No Notes:
Conflict of Interest: Are the relationships (personal/financial, etc.) of the guideline developers fully disclosed?	Yes/No Notes:

IOM STANDARD	IS THE STANDARD MET?
Group Composition: Do the credentials of the guideline developers represent a diverse group of expertise?	Yes/No Notes:
Systematic Review: Is there a process for methodical review of evidence identified?	Yes/No Notes:
Rating of Recommendations: Is there a system for rating the recommendations and is it described?	Yes/No Notes:
Articulation of Recommendations: Are the recommendations clear?	Yes/No Notes:
External Review: Is the process for external review sound?	Yes/No Notes:
Updating: Is the guideline reviewed and updated?	Yes/No Notes:

IOM, Institute of Medicine.

In your own words, describe how this guideline is related to:

Population of interest:

Problem of interest:

1. Describe three specific recommendations in the guideline that are related to your problem:

   1.

   2.

   3.

Do you think this guideline is being following in clinical practice?

List the potential barriers and facilitators of guideline use:

BARRIERS	FACILITATORS

SUMMARY

The purpose of a CPG is to reduce variation in practice. However, guidelines do not replace the importance of critical thinking and individualization of patient care (Christenbery, 2018). When you have identified an agency/organization to partner with for your project, further explore the protocols and clinical guidelines used in the institution to consider how they impact your project. Next steps:

- Explore the partnering organization's use of guidelines, protocols, and pathways.
- If there is more than one guideline relevant to the same problem, use the AGREE II Instrument to compare them (www.agreetrust.org/agree-ii/).

REFERENCES AND RESOURCES

American Association of Colleges of Nursing. (2015). *The doctor of nursing practice: Current issues and clarifying recommendations.* https://www.aacnnursing.org/Portals/42/News/White-Papers/DNP-Implementation-TF-Report-8-15.pdf

Appraisal of Guidelines for Research & Evaluation II. (2017). *AGREE II instrument.* https://www.agreetrust.org/wp-content/uploads/2017/12/AGREE-II-Users-Manual-and-23-item-Instrument-2009-Update-2017.pdf

Christenbery, T. (Ed.). (2018). *Evidence-based practice in nursing.* Springer Publishing Company.

Institute of Medicine. (2011). *Clinical practice guidelines we can trust.* National Academies Press. http://data.care-statement.org/wp-content/uploads/2016/12/IOMGuidelines-2013-1.pdf

RELATED TEXTBOOK

Christenbery, T. (Ed.). (2018). *Evidence-based practice in nursing.* Springer Publishing Company.
 Chapter 9: Clinical Practice Guidelines

LESSON 4.5

POLICIES RELATED TO THE PROBLEM

BACKGROUND

Now that you have identified a problem, it is important to consider how health policy fits into the picture. It is also important to remember that most of what we do and how we practice are guided, in some way, by health policy. This may include local, state, or national policies, but clearly there is an impetus behind why we do what we do that is grounded in health policy. This means that it is important that nurses, especially doctorally prepared nurses, are not merely reacting to the health policy, but rather play an active role in developing and evaluating health policy.

"Nurses must see policy as something they can shape rather than something that happens to them."
—Institute of Medicine (IOM, 2011), *The Future of Nursing: Leading Change, Advancing Health*

The American Association of Colleges of Nursing's (AACN, 2006) Essential V outlines how the DNP graduate can influence healthcare policy through advocacy in healthcare. Consider the reach of health policy and its influences on health disparities, ethics, access to and quality of care, and equity and social justice. Being aware and taking an active role in advocating for health policy issues is part of being a responsible nurse leader and is necessary as part of our professional practice. Remember, these policies are guiding the way we practice; therefore, we should not only be aware, but we should have a voice and seat at the table. The IOM (2011) also reminds us that DNP graduates can frame healthcare financing, practice regulation, access, safety, quality, and efficacy of care through their ability to design, influence, and implement healthcare policies.

Never underestimate your ability to influence health policy on any level. Your DNP education has provided you with the skills to be leaders and advocates who can not only advance your own practice but also protect your patients.

LEARNING OBJECTIVES

- Learners will be able to analyze their own contribution to health policy.
- Learners will be able to identify existing health policy pertaining to their problem of interest.

ACTIVITIES

Understanding Your Contribution to Health Policy

As a novice DNP nurse, you are able to review the literature and research supporting certain health policies. As a result, you are able to develop a new and unique awareness of issues of which you may have previously been unaware. This eye-opening exposure is the first step in recognizing your potential to influence policy. As you become more knowledgeable about the health policy process, you can increase your involvement in issues important to you and be a contributor to health policy.

ORGANIZATION	ISSUES/EFFORTS	RESULT
Example: Student representative on university's School of Nursing curriculum committee (*local influencer*)	• Need for reevaluation due to student evaluations/updated DNP requirements/variations across programs • Have an active voice in providing student perspectives on course sequencing, concurrent courses, facilitators/challenges, and course deliverables	• Awareness of process and influencers on curriculum development within the school • Input on institutional policy for curriculum plans of study
Local organizational influencer		
State organizational influencer		
National organizational influencer		

✅ **Consider your problem of interest. Is there any existing health policy associated with this problem?** Consider larger pieces of work that can also impact the problem of interest, including IOM reports, Centers for Medicare & Medicaid Services guidelines/requirements, Joint Commission Standards, and so on. Complete the following table. Be concise. Write one to two sentences for each item.

Problem of Interest:

Organizational policy	
State policy	
National policy	

SUMMARY

The goal of this lesson is to allow you to consider how you can influence health policy. This lesson also allows you to focus on how your problem of interest is influenced by health policy at various levels. Reflect with your faculty or DNP chair on what you have identified about how your project is influencing or being influenced by health policy.

REFERENCES AND RESOURCES

American Association of Colleges of Nursing. (2006). *The essentials of doctoral education for advanced nursing practice.* https://www.aacnnursing.org/Portals/42/Publications/DNPEssentials.pdf

Institute of Medicine. (2001). *Crossing the quality chasm: A new health system for the 21st century*. National Academies Press.

Institute of Medicine. (2011). *The future of nursing: Leading change, advancing health*. National Academies Press.

RELATED TEXTBOOKS

Hickey, J. V., & Brosnan, C. A. (Eds.). (2017). *Evaluation of healthcare quality for the DNP* (2nd ed.). Springer Publishing Company.

   Chapter 13: Translating Outcomes From Evaluation to Health Policy

Zalon, M., & Patton, R. (2018). *Nurses making policy* (2nd ed.). Springer Publishing Company.

   Unit II: Analyzing Policy

   Chapter 4: Identifying a Problem and Analyzing a Policy Issue

   Chapter 5: Harnessing Evidence in the Policy Process

LESSON 4.6

USING THE QUADRUPLE AIM TO EXAMINE THE PROBLEM

BACKGROUND

The Institute for Healthcare Improvement (IHI) advocates for the Triple Aim. The Triple Aim describes a goal. It states that healthcare should work toward (a) improving the patient experience, (b) improving the health of populations, and (c) reducing the cost of healthcare (IHI, 2019). Recently, a fourth goal has been added (IHI, 2017). It asserts that to care for patients, we, the healthcare team, must also care for ourselves (Bodenheimer & Sinsky, 2014). Thus, the Triple Aim is now being referred to as the *Quadruple Aim* (Figure 4.3). In this lesson, we use this IHI model to examine the relationship of these goals to your problem of interest.

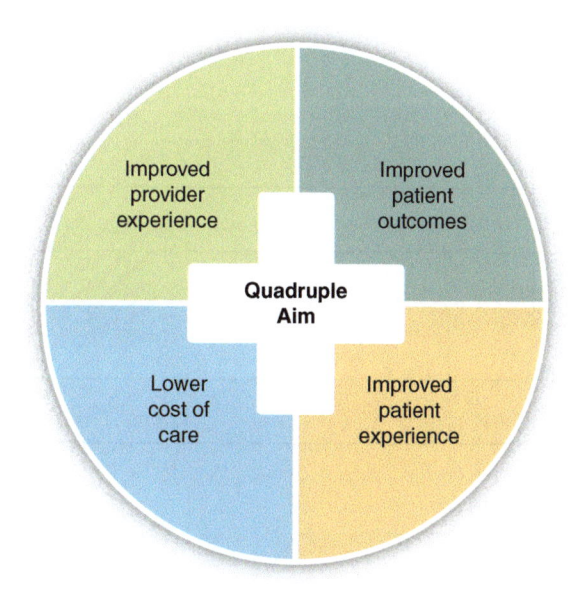

Figure 4.3 The Quadruple Aim.

LEARNING OBJECTIVES

- List factors that impact the problem of interest.
- Explore the relationships between the problem of interest and the Quadruple Aim.

ACTIVITIES

Under each column, list key points, information, and facts related to the problem of interest.

COST	POPULATION HEALTH	PATIENT EXPERIENCE	PROVIDER EXPERIENCE
What are the issues related to cost for both the system and the patients?	What are the issues that impact the collective health of the population?	What are the issues related to patient satisfaction? What are the issues related to quality of care and safety of the patients?	What are the issues that impact the healthcare providers and healthcare team?

In reflecting on this information, how does it collectively relate to your problem of interest?

_____

_____

_____

What are the key takeaway points?

Takeaway 1:

_____

_____

_____

Takeaway 2:

_____

_____

_____

NEXT STEPS

- Talk to your DNP faculty about your findings.
- Continue to talk to colleagues and organizational stakeholders.

REFERENCES AND RESOURCES

Bodenheimer, T., & Sinsky, C. (2014). From triple to Quadruple Aim: Care of the patient requires care of the provider. *The Annals of Family Medicine, 12*(6), 573–576.

Institute for Healthcare Improvement [Screen name]. (2017, November 28). *IHI's position on the Quadruple Aim.* [Video file]. https://youtu.be/d1uX0WFcAY

Institute for Healthcare Improvement. (2019). *The IHI Triple Aim.* https://www.marquette.edu/center-for-teaching-and-learning/interprofessional-education.php

> **RELATED TEXTBOOK**
>
> Hickey, J. V., & Brosnan, C. A. (2017). *Evaluation of health care quality for DNPs* (2nd ed.). Springer Publishing Company.
> Chapter 5: Economic Evaluation
> Chapter 6: Evaluation of Organizations
> Chapter 7: Evaluation of Healthcare Information Systems and Patient Care
> Chapter 11: Healthcare Teams

LESSON 4.7

IMPACT OF THE PROBLEM ON PATIENTS, FAMILIES, AND COMMUNITIES: SOCIAL DETERMINANTS OF HEALTH

BACKGROUND

At the heart of nursing is a desire to serve our patients, their families, and communities. The problems they experience provide a starting point to initiate change. Our goal in this exercise is to fully explore the impact of a problem on these entities through the lens of social determinants of health (Healthy People, n.d.-c).

To start, consider talking to people. Talk to your patients about how their health problems affect them. Remember, you are trying to understand, not to collect official project data. What challenges do they have navigating the health system? How does their family cope? In the literature, you may identify qualitative research studies that will help you. Qualitative research helps to describe the lived experiences of patients and families. For example, what is it like to experience fatigue with multiple sclerosis? Try to better understand your problem of interest from a patient's perspective. Then, try to relate to their family.

To better assess community, Healthy People (n.d.-a, n.d.-b) offers a framework called "MAP-IT" (**M**obilize, **A**ssess, **P**lan, **I**mplement, **T**rack). We use their suggested activities under "assess" to ensure that you are fully examining the impact of your problem of interest on the community. The tools will also help you set priorities.

LEARNING OBJECTIVES

- Outline the impact of the problem on patients.
- Trace the impact of the problem on the patient's family.
- Report the impact of the problem on the larger community.

ACTIVITIES

Impact on Patients

Use qualitative literature or personal communications to answer the following questions:

- How does the problem impact your activities of daily living?
- How does the problem impact your coping ability?
- How does the problem impact your finances?
- How does the problem impact your spirituality?
- How does the problem impact your relationships with others?
- What is the most difficult thing about your condition/problem/diagnosis?
- Is there anything about the situation that could be improved?

Impact on Families

Use qualitative literature or personal communications to answer the following questions:

- How does the problem impact your relationship with your family member?
- What challenges do you personally have with the situation?
- Is there anything about the situation that could be improved?

Impact on Community

Consider the impact of the problem on the community to answer these questions:

- Who is affected and how?
- What resources do we have in the community?
- What resources do we need in the community?

☑ To pull these concepts together, consider the Healthy People 2020 social determinants of health (Healthy People, n.d.-c). How do the five social determinants of health mentioned in Healthy People impact your problem?

1. Economic stability:

_____

_____

2. Education:
_____
_____

3. Social and community context:
_____
_____

4. Health and healthcare:
_____
_____
_____

5. Neighborhood and built environment:
_____
_____

Explore additional resources on community assessment for more detailed analysis.

NEXT STEPS

- Explore additional resources on community assessment for more detailed analysis.
- Summarize and organize your findings for later use.

REFERENCES AND RESOURCES

CDC, CHANGE Tool. (n.d.). *Building a foundation of knowledge to prioritize community needs: An action guide.* https://www.cdc.gov/nccdphp/dch/programs/healthycommunitiesprogram/tools/change/pdf/changeactionguide.pdf

Community Tool Box. (n.d.). *Chapter 3: Assessing community needs and resources.* https://ctb.ku.edu/en/table-of-contents/assessment/assessing-community-needs-and-resources

Healthy People. (n.d.-a). *MAP-IT framework: ASSESS.* https://www.healthypeople.gov/2020/tools-and-resources/program-planning/Assess

Healthy People. (n.d.-b). *Program planning: MAP IT framework.* https://www.healthypeople.gov/2020/tools-and-resources/Program-Planning

Healthy People. (n.d.-c). *Social determinants of health.* https://www.healthypeople.gov/2020/topics-objectives/topic/social-determinants-of-health

RELATED TEXTBOOK

Hickey, J. V., & Brosnan, C. A. (2017). *Evaluation of health care quality for DNPs* (2nd ed.). Springer Publishing Company.
- Chapter 8: Program Evaluation
- Chapter 12: Evaluation of Populations and Population Health

LESSON 4.8

IMPACT OF THE PROBLEM ON ORGANIZATIONS

BACKGROUND

Although you have been focusing on understanding the problem and its impact on others, it is just as important to be aware of how the problem impacts the organization and how to properly assess an organization in order to facilitate improvements. Keep in mind that if the problem is not a priority for the organization, you will likely face many roadblocks in your ability to successfully implement your project.

Understanding the organization and the impact of the problem on it is necessary in order to obtain buy-in from the organization and recognition of the importance of the problem. The first step is to properly assess the organization and analyze workflow. This includes systematically reviewing key indicators, requiring all parts of the organization to work together, and recognizing the need for resources and support (Hickey & Brosnan, 2017). This requires you to think not only internally about the unit in which you plan to conduct your project but also about the larger organization. Our goal in this exercise is to look at the impact of the problem through the lens of a nurse leader.

First, understand the organization. Recognize that depending on your role within the organization, there is more going on than you may realize. What do you know about the organization? What type of organization is it? How does it generate revenue? What is the reach of the organization? For example, what is the size and location of the organization and how does that impact the type and scope of services it provides? A small, community-based hospital that offers routine obstetrical services and low-risk deliveries may rely on referral services for high-risk obstetrical care rather than treat in-house. As a result, a project focusing on the preeclamptic patient may not be feasible at this organization.

You will also want to understand the leadership structure and mission/vision/values of the organization. Having an understanding of the decision-makers and the fundamental beliefs driving the organization is also important, as they guide how decisions are made and where to focus efforts. If an organization's mission is to serve the underprivileged, certainly a project that looks to address this would at least pique its interest. Who are the players who make decisions? Certainly the C-suite, but who else? Specific to your project, you will want to know who oversees projects/research. Including them is pertinent and necessary. Knowing what initiatives are on their radar will also help identify whether your problem is equally as important to them.

Once you have completed an organizational assessment, you will conduct a workflow analysis, which will ensure that the outcomes you were hoping for actually occur. Depending on the nature of your project, this may include productivity or efficiency in the process, customer/patient satisfaction, compliance, and even employee engagement. It's important to recognize that workflow analysis is the review of how the work *actually* gets done, not the protocols/methods in place that guide how it *should* be done.

According to the Agency for Healthcare Research and Quality (AHRQ, 2015), redesigning workflows has two goals: (a) improving performance and (b) increasing efficiency. After you outline actual practice, you can then work with other stakeholders in redesigning the workflow to incorporate the desired improvements/processes and then test these changes.

LEARNING OBJECTIVES

- Identify key components of the organizational structure and basic factors influencing decision-making efforts.
- Utilize workflow analysis to identify opportunities for improvement in care delivery processes.

ACTIVITIES

Conduct an organizational assessment of the intended project site. Use these prompts based on the content outlined by Hickey and Brosnan (2017), Table 6.1, Key Components of Organization and System Evaluation.

The Basics of the Organization

ORGANIZATIONAL COMPONENT	NOTES
History and overview	
Type of organization	
Funding/revenue sources	
Governance	
Mission, vision, and values	
Strategy and goals	
Size and scope of services	
Culture	
Organizational structure	
Authority and decision-making	
Reputation	
Outcomes, quality, and patient satisfaction	
Role of nursing	

Does the organization agree that your problem of interest is a priority?

_____

_____

What is the gap in this organization? Why is this problem occurring? What does the organization want to improve?

_____

_____

_____

_____

✓ **Within organizations, there are complex processes. Workflow analysis is a broad process and might include looking at the flow of a patient who is transitioning, the process of prescribing and filling a medication, or the flow of information between healthcare team members. List three workflows or processes related to your problem or population of interest.**

1.

2.

3.

Now, select the process that is most likely to have the biggest impact on your problem or population. Review the Institute for Healthcare Improvement (IHI) content on improving workflow and removing waste, available at www.ihi.org/resources/Pages/Changes/ImproveWorkFlowandRemoveWaste.aspx. Then, read through the content on workflow redesign from the HealthIT.gov website (www.healthit.gov/faq/what-workflow-redesign-why-it-important).

On a separate sheet of paper, complete a workflow analysis of the identified problem using one of the suggested tools:

- Root-cause analysis
- https://videos.asq.org/asking-why-with-root-cause-and-5-whys
- https://asq.org/quality-resources/root-cause-analysis
- AHRQ (2015)
- https://pcmh.ahrq.gov/sites/default/files/attachments/pcpf-module-10-workflow-mapping.pdf
- Other:

NEXT STEPS

- Discuss your findings with stakeholders and your faculty.
- Take note of opportunities for improvement that you identify.

REFERENCES AND RESOURCES

Agency for Healthcare Research and Quality. (2015). *Primary care practice facilitation curriculum. Module 10: Mapping and redesigning workflow.* https://pcmh.ahrq.gov/sites/default/files/attachments/pcpf-module-10-workflow-mapping.pdf

Hickey, J. V., & Brosnan, C. A. (Eds.). (2017). *Evaluation of health care quality for DNPs* (2nd ed.). Springer Publishing Company.

RELATED TEXTBOOK

Hickey, J. V., & Brosnan, C. A. (Eds.). (2017). *Evaluation of health care quality for DNPs* (2nd ed.). Springer Publishing Company.
- Chapter 6: Evaluation of Organizations and Systems
- Chapter 7: Evaluation of Health Care Information Systems and Patient Care Technology
- Chapter 8: Program Evaluation
- Chapter 9: Quality Improvement

LESSON 4.9

DEMONSTRATING THE VALUE OF THE DNP PROJECT

BACKGROUND

As you approach stakeholders, you will need to be able to provide an overview of what might be done to solve the problem. "Might" is the optimal word because at this point, a formal review of literature has not been completed to find evidence supporting your proposed intervention. In the first exercise, we will help you think about possible interventions from a broad perspective. According to the Institute of Medicine (IOM), education alone as an intervention will change practice only 4% of the time (IOM, 2011). Therefore, we recommend that you think beyond just "educating" on a topic.

Stakeholders will also want to know what value your project brings. Value to the population. Value to the agency. Value to the larger healthcare system. In the final activity of this lesson, you will utilize the Value Pyramid to consider the possibilities.

LEARNING OBJECTIVES

- Consider the value added by the DNP Project.
- Demonstrate the project value to stakeholders.

ACTIVITIES

Interventions and solutions to improve health outcomes should be evidence based. White et al. (2020) discuss the top methods for evidence translation. Review the information in this table and highlight the three methods that could work best in the context of your DNP Project.

Academic detailing	Audit and feedback	Bundles	Decision support	Order sets
Practice guidelines	Process redesign	Protocols	Quality improvement	Scorecards and dashboards
Teaming	Technology-based solutions	Tool kits (practice resources)	Other:	Other:

Three possibilities for my project are:

1.

2.

3.

In the next activity, we will need to consider the value your project brings. A DNP Project must be valued by an organization, population, or entity. Review the 30 Elements of Value shown in Figure 4.4. According to the author, the more the elements of value are added, the better the product or services. (Read more at: https://hbr.org/2016/09/the-elements-of-value.)

List five elements from Figure 4.4 that your DNP Project could add:

1.

2.

3.

4.

5.

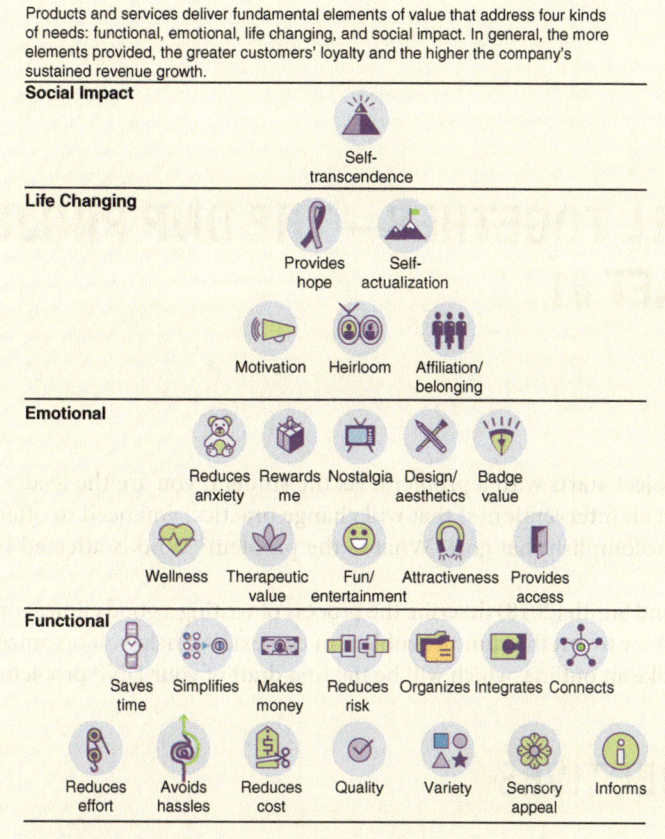

Figure 4.4 The elements of value pyramid.
Source: Almquist, E., Senior, J., & Bloch, N. (2016). The elements of value. *Harvard Business Review, 94*(9), 47–53.

NEXT STEPS

- Review this information with your faculty.
- Determine your most viable project options.
- Begin to search for literature documenting interventions others have done to achieve the outcomes you want to achieve.

REFERENCES AND RESOURCES

Almquist, E., Senior, J., & Bloch, N. (2016). The elements of value. *Harvard Business Review, 94*(9), 47–53.
Institute of Medicine. (2011). *Clinical practice guidelines we can trust*. National Academies Press.
White, K. M., Dudley-Brown, S., & Terhaar, M. F. (Eds.). (2020). *Translation of evidence into nursing and healthcare* (3rd ed.). Springer Publishing Company.

RELATED TEXTBOOK

White, K. M., Dudley-Brown, S., & Terhaar, M. F. (Eds.). (2020). *Translation of evidence into nursing and healthcare* (3rd ed.). Springer Publishing Company.

Chapter 4: Translation of Evidence to Improve Clinical Outcomes

Chapter 5: Translation of Evidence for Improving Safety and Quality

Chapter 6: Translation of Evidence for Leadership

Chapter 7: Translation of Evidence for Health Policy

Chapter 8: Methods for Translation

LESSON 4.10

PUTTING IT ALL TOGETHER—THE DNP PROJECT OUTLINE: DRAFT #1

BACKGROUND

The DNP Project starts with a problem. As the student, you are the leader of the DNP team. In order to implement an intervention(s) that will change practice, you need to offer a proposal describing how you plan to accomplish that goal. What is the problem? Who is affected by the problem? Why is it a problem?

Bonnel and Smith (2018) describe the process of writing a good clinical problem statement. They offer strategies on how to put the clinical problem in context. We help you organize your information from this chapter to make an outline, which will be the first draft of your DNP problem statement and background.

LEARNING OBJECTIVES

- Prepare a draft of the DNP problem statement.
- Outline the elements of the background for the DNP Project proposal.

ACTIVITIES

Reflect on the information that you have gathered about your problem of interest. Begin to narrow and funnel the information to focus the problem.

Problem of interest:

Population it impacts:

I know it is a problem because: (List your top three key points from your gathering of information.)

1.

2.

3.

Why is it important to address this problem?

Now, put this information into a sentence format. Example:

_____ (condition/disease) _____ is a significant health problem for _____ (population of interest) _____. _____ (key point #1) _____, _____ (key point #2) _____, and _____ (key point #3) _____ are all factors that contribute to the problem. As a result, these patients experience negative health outcomes, such as _____ (outcome #1) _____ and _____ (outcome #2) _____.

> **Example:**
>
> "COPD is a significant health problem for Kentucky residents. Tobacco abuse, medication noncompliance, and poor self-management of the disease are all factors that contribute to the problem. As a result, these patients experience negative health outcomes such as hospitalization and decreased quality of life."

Write a draft of your final problem statement:

- ☐ Did you state the problem? (What is the problem?)
- ☐ Did you identify the population of interest? (Who is affected?)
- ☐ Did you include key points that contribute to the problem? (Why is it a problem?)
- ☐ Did you identify the outcomes that need improvement?

Outline the first draft of your DNP Project proposal in context using the information you have collected. Refer to your school's requirements and discuss with your faculty before you begin. Modify as required.

DNP Project Outline: Draft #1

Title page

Abstract (always written last, hold a spot but skip this for now)

Introduction

Background

- Problem of interest
- Population of interest
- Relevant definition(s)
- Results of initial inquiries and searches: demographics, incidence, and prevalence
- Strategic agendas related to the problem
- Policies related to the problem
- Clinical guidelines related to the problem
- Quadruple aim
- Impact on patients, families, and community: social determinant of health
- Impact on healthcare systems and organizations
- Desired outcomes and potential solutions
- Value added by the DNP Project

Remember to consult with your faculty and review the DNP Project proposal guidelines for your school. Students often ask, "How long should a DNP Project proposal be?" This cannot be consistently quantified. We would *roughly* suggest one to two paragraphs for each component in the preceding list depending on the situation. Additional content may be needed. Seek help early in the writing process. Get someone to proofread what you write. Remember that many people will read this document, so you have to explain things, provide definitions, and make the sections flow logically.

NEXT STEPS

- Present your problem statement and outline to your faculty.
- Discuss and finalize the project goals and desired outcomes.

REFERENCE AND RESOURCE

Bonnel, W., & Smith, K. (2018). *Proposal writing for clinical nursing and DNP Projects*. Springer Publishing Company.

> **RELATED TEXTBOOK**
>
> Bonnel, W., & Smith, K. (2018). *Proposal writing for clinical nursing and DNP Projects*. Springer Publishing Company.
> Chapter 1: Introduction: Why a Scholarly Proposal for the Clinical Project Proposal?
> Chapter 2: Using the Writing Plan as a Developmental Tool for the Advanced Clinical Project
> Chapter 3: Writing a Good Clinical Problem Statement and Placing the Clinical Problem in Context

CHAPTER SUMMARY

The purpose of this chapter was to fully investigate your problem of interest:

- What is the problem?
- Who is affected by the problem?
- Why is it a problem?

Briefly you began to explore

- Where is this problem occurring (context)?
- What needs to be improved?
- How could it be improved?

You have gathered information, prepared a problem statement, outlined content for the background of the proposal, and considered your desired outcomes for the project. The next step depends on the layout of your DNP curriculum. The order of Chapter 5, Skills for Formal Review of Literature and Evidence Appraisal and Chapter 6, Framing the DNP Project—Taking Aim and Being SMART could be interchanged. After consultation with your faculty, your next goal will be to

- Complete a formal review of literature on a focused question (Chapter 5).
- Frame the project using defined aims and objectives (Chapter 6).

OR

- Frame the project using defined aims and objectives (Chapter 6).
- Complete a formal review of literature on a focused question (Chapter 5).

Reflections

What are two things you have learned in this chapter?

1.

2.

What questions or concerns do you still have at this point? How will you reconcile them?

1.

2.

Be open-minded. DNP Projects evolve. The project may take shape in a way that you did not originally consider. These are real-world projects with real-world problems. Stay the course and communicate with your faculty. Don't spend too much time in your own mind. Involve your DNP team. Seek information beyond this workbook using the suggested resources and reading the suggested Springer Publishing Company texts.
Continue to work hard!

NOTES

5

Review of Literature, Evidence Appraisal, and PICO Question Development

Editor: Aaron M. Sebach
Contributors: Molly Bradshaw, Tracy R. Vitale, Margaret Dreker, Irina Benenson, and Marilyn Oermann

Lessons

Lesson 5.1 Types of Evidence and Literature Reviews

Lesson 5.2 Formalizing a PICO Question

Lesson 5.3 Selecting Appropriate Databases

Lesson 5.4 Documenting Your Search, Annotation, and Citation Management

Lesson 5.5 Options for Evidence Appraisal

Lesson 5.6 Appraisal, Comparison, and Reconciliation of Clinical Practice Guidelines

Lesson 5.7 Constructing an Evidence Table

Lesson 5.8 Synthesizing the Evidence

OBJECTIVES

Review and appraisal of literature is an important skill for DNP students and, ultimately, DNP-prepared nurses. A formal literature review is a well-defined process wherein a specific question is formulated, a methodical literature search is completed, and findings are documented, appraised, and communicated. By the end of this chapter, you will be able to

- Develop a clinical question using the PICO (patient/problem, intervention, comparison, outcome) format.
- Complete a literature review and document your search.
- Explore options for evidence appraisal.
- Construct an evidence table.
- Write a synthesis of findings from your literature review.

INTRODUCTION

At this point, you have identified a clinical problem and population of interest for your DNP Project. Your problem statement, incorporating your identified clinical problem and population of interest, will provide a foundation for your work in this chapter. You are encouraged to make your problem statement the wallpaper on your computer and/or post it on the bulletin board in your office. Doing so will keep your problem statement at the forefront of your work, maintaining your focus. Now that you have a solid understanding of the background and context of your identified clinical problem, it is time to ask more focused questions through an appraisal of the evidence.

Reviewing and appraising evidence is a refined skill. While gathering background information in Chapters 3 and 4, you explored the literature and supporting evidence. However, it is unlikely that you utilized a formal process. Rather, you gathered information to understand your identified clinical problem. Now, you should begin to think about what else you need to know. Do you need to know more about a certain outcome? Do you need to know more about evidence-based solutions to improve that outcome? Do you need to know more about how to evaluate or measure identified intervention(s)? Write down what else you need to know. You will return to this list of questions when conducting your literature review. This is an important step in the process, so take your time. Collaborate with your faculty, clinical partners, and mentor(s).

In this chapter, you will hone a spirit of inquiry (Melnyk et al., 2019) and develop the requisite skills for scholarly inquiry. For purposes of this workbook, the phrase "formal review of literature" refers to a pointed strategy for developing a clinical question, searching the literature, appraising the literature, and making sense of the findings. You will learn the different types of literature reviews and their working definitions. Your school may have requirements regarding the type of literature review required for your DNP program.

There will be one overarching question that drives your project and inquiry process. Familiarize yourself with the skills required to develop a question, search and appraise the literature, and synthesize your findings. Then work with your faculty, clinical partners, and mentor(s) to determine their best fit to your project while meeting the requirements established by your school.

Keep in mind that this chapter offers a general overview. Therefore, it is essential that you develop and maintain relationships with librarians and other colleagues before and during your literature review. Additional training beyond coursework is often required, especially for completion of systematic reviews using Cochrane or Joanna Briggs Institute methodologies (Cochrane, n.d.; Joanna Briggs Institute, n.d.). Finally, it is important to note that your DNP Project will not be an integrative or systematic review. DNP Projects require implementation of a clinical practice change based on the evidence. The heart of DNP scholarship is translation of evidence to practice.

REFERENCES AND RESOURCES

Cochrane. (n.d.). *Cochrane training*. https://training.cochrane.org
Joanna Briggs Institute. (n.d.). *Education*. https://jbi.global/education
Melnyk, B. M., Fineout-Overholt, E., Stillwell, S. B., & Williamson, K. M. (2019). *Evidence based practice: A step by step guide. Igniting a spirit of inquiry*. http://forces4quality.org/af4q/download-document/3517/Resource-Evidence_Based_Practice__Step_by_Step__Igniting_a.28.pdf

RELATED TEXTBOOK

Holly, C., Salmond, S., & Saimbert, M. (Eds.). (2021). *Comprehensive systematic review for advanced practice nursing* (3rd ed.). Springer Publishing Company.

MY GOALS FOR SKILLS FOR FORMAL REVIEW OF THE LITERATURE AND EVIDENCE APPRAISAL ARE TO:

1.
2.
3.

LESSON 5.1

TYPES OF EVIDENCE AND LITERATURE REVIEWS

BACKGROUND

Fundamentally, evidence is credible information generated from research studies designed to answer questions or describe a phenomenon of interest. As a DNP student, you are charged with appraising the quality of research studies and determining the applicability to practice. Your ultimate goal is to translate the best evidence to practice (Christenbery, 2017).

LEARNING OBJECTIVES

- Identify primary versus secondary literature.
- Differentiate quantitative and qualitative research.
- Examine the evidence pyramid.
- Articulate the differences in types of literature reviews.

ACTIVITIES

There are different types of literature. Review the following terms:

- **Primary literature**: an original experiment or firsthand account describing a phenomenon; sometimes called a "primary study."
- **Secondary literature**: a summary or synthesis of primary literature; for example, meta-analysis or meta-synthesis.
- **Tertiary literature**: a summary of primary and secondary literature; for example, a textbook.
- **Filtered literature**: literature that is reviewed and pooled to explore common outcomes in similar circumstances (Holly et al., 2021).

☑ Literature is organized by the type of research study: quantitative, qualitative, or mixed method. Mixed method studies incorporate both qualitative and quantitative data. To understand differences between quantitative and qualitative research, review the following table.

QUANTITATIVE RESEARCH	QUALITATIVE RESEARCH
Purpose: describe, explain, predict, and determine the probability of cause–effect relationships	Purpose: describe, explore, discover, and seek understanding of phenomena
Research designs: descriptive, correlational, quasi-experimental, experimental	Research designs: ethnography, phenomenology, grounded theory, case study, narrative inquiry, historical review
Measurements: numerical data that can be statistically analyzed	Measurements: nonnumerical data (e.g., words, images, and artifacts) that are manually analyzed

Source: Data from Christenbery, T. (2017). *Evidence-based practice in nursing.* Springer Publishing Company.

Evidence is often visually organized into an evidence pyramid (Figure 5.1). Information higher on the pyramid is often more compelling. Observational (qualitative) studies form the pyramid's foundation, followed by experiential (quantitative) studies. At the top, there is filtered or synthesized information. As you critically appraise the evidence, your final clinical practice change recommendation will be based on multiple studies.

REFLECTION

- Where do background information and expert opinion fall on the pyramid? Think of these as the information you gathered for the project background. Now, you need to ask a more specific question and identify the best evidence to answer that question.
- The question you ask will often determine the type of evidence you find. Based on your question, do you anticipate finding more observational (qualitative) studies or experimental (quantitative) studies?

A literature review involves the process of collecting pieces of evidence to answer a specific question. Consider the differences between the review types in the table following Figure 5.1.

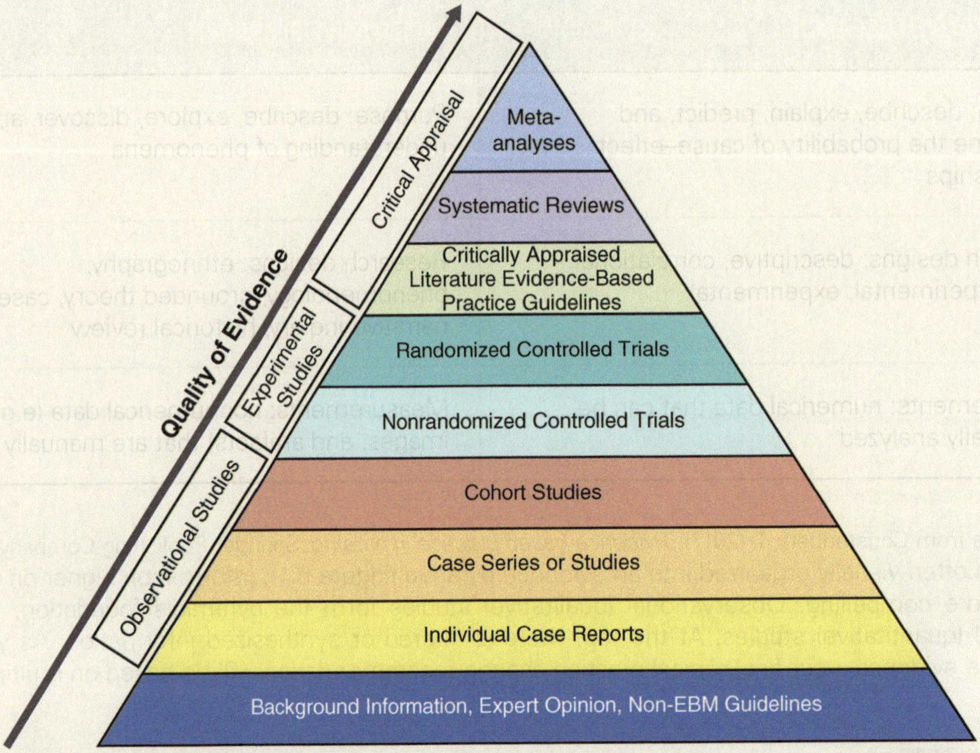
Meta-analyses
Systematic Reviews
Critically Appraised Literature Evidence-Based Practice Guidelines
Randomized Controlled Trials
Nonrandomized Controlled Trials
Cohort Studies
Case Series or Studies
Individual Case Reports
Background Information, Expert Opinion, Non-EBM Guidelines
Quality of Evidence
Critical Appraisal
Experimental Studies
Observational Studies

Figure 5.1 The evidence pyramid. EBM, evidence-based medicine.
Source: Central Michigan University. (n.d.). *Evidence-based medicine: Resources by levels of evidence.* https://libguides.cmich.edu/cmed/ebm/pyramid

	FORMAL LITERATURE REVIEW	INTEGRATIVE REVIEW	SYSTEMATIC REVIEW
Focus	**Broad**	**Defined**	**Precise**
Search Strategy	Based on keywords; search two to three databases and limit to the past 5 years	Based on keywords and MeSH terms; searches for pivotal papers (research or theory) in two to six databases or search engines	Exhaustive, including hand searches and searches for unpublished (grey) literature; uses an explicit strategy
Appraisal	Rapid appraisal, if any; is performed to establish support for the question Recommendations by: The Ohio State University and Johns Hopkins Medicine	May be rigorous; generally done by one reviewer Recommendations by: Toronto & Remington (2020)	Rigorous; completed by two independent reviewers; uses valid and reliable tools for appraisal based on the design of the study Recommendations by: Cochrane and Joanna Briggs Institute

(continued)

	FORMAL LITERATURE REVIEW	**INTEGRATIVE REVIEW**	**SYSTEMATIC REVIEW**
Focus	**Broad**	**Defined**	**Precise**
Outcome	Support; not generally considered a good source for clinical decision-making	Offers a recommendation; selected literature should be analyzed, not just summarized; articles and groups of articles are compared, themes are identified, and gaps are noted	Suggests a best practice; the purpose of a systematic review is to reach a conclusion regarding a topic: e.g., the selection of high-quality studies to be used in a meta-analysis, the gaps in current research, or the best clinical evidence for determining evidence-based practice
DNP Project Considerations	Answers a question, supports some component of the DNP Project, and is more focused than the project background	Answers a question, makes project-related recommendations, and should be rigorous	Answers a question, precisely articulates best practice, and is rigorous

MeSH, Medical Subject Headings.

Source: Adapted from Holly, C. (2019). *Practice-based scholarly inquiry and the DNP Project.* Springer Publishing Company.

Expert Commentary: Marilyn Oermann, PhD, RN, ANEF, FAAN

There are many different types of reviews of research and literature that you can do. Three common types are systematic, integrative, and literature (or narrative) reviews. Use of these terms varies, but all reviews answer questions or describe what is known (and gaps) about a topic. The goal of a systematic review is to answer a specific clinical or research question by carefully searching for and selecting studies based on predetermined criteria and critically appraising them. Systematic reviews use an explicit and reproducible methodology for searching relevant bibliographic databases, such as MEDLINE and Cumulative Index to Nursing and Allied Health Literature (CINAHL); including selected studies in the review; evaluating the quality of individual studies; and synthesizing the findings. With some systematic reviews, the researchers also do a meta-analysis, which uses statistical techniques to integrate the results.

Integrative reviews are broad reviews that include both research and theoretical literature. Because of the various types of studies in these reviews, they provide a more comprehensive summary of a topic than a systematic review, which is focused on answering a specific question. An integrative review includes various types of literature, making it difficult to critically appraise studies as done in a systematic review. A literature review, which is a narrative review, searches for current information on a topic to reveal what is known and gaps in our understanding.

Each of these reviews follows a carefully planned and documented search strategy, which outlines the Medical Subject Headings (MeSH) and key terms and phrases used for the search, variations of search terms, combinations, bibliographic databases searched, and results of the search. You should consult with a librarian to develop the search strategy for your project.

NEXT STEPS

- Think about the question you want to answer.
- Consider what type(s) of evidence will support the question/intervention/outcome.
- Collaborate with your faculty on the best approach to your literature review.
- If you select an integrative review, utilize the Toronto and Remington (2020) text to guide your work.

REFERENCES AND RESOURCES

Central Michigan University. (n.d.). *Evidence-based medicine: Resources by levels of evidence.* https://libguides.cmich.edu/cmed/ebm/pyramid

Christenbery, T. (Ed.). (2017). *Evidence-based practice in nursing.* Springer Publishing Company.

Cochrane. (n.d.). *Cochrane training.* https://training.cochrane.org

Holly, C. (2019). *Practice-based scholarly inquiry and the DNP project.* Springer Publishing Company.

Holly, C., Salmond, S., & Saimbert, M. (Eds.). (2021). *Comprehensive systematic review for advanced practice nursing* (3rd ed.). Springer Publishing Company.

Joanna Briggs Institute. (n.d.). *Education.* https://jbi.global/education

Johns Hopkins Medicine. (n.d.). *Center for evidence-based practice.* https://www.hopkinsmedicine.org/evidence-based-practice/

The Ohio State University. (n.d.). *Helene Fuld health trust national institute for evidence-based practice in nursing and healthcare.* https://fuld.nursing.osu.edu/

Toronto, C. E., & Remington, R. (Eds.). (2020). *A step-by-step guide to conducting an integrative review.* Springer Publishing Company.

RELATED TEXTBOOKS

Christenbery, T. (Ed.). (2017). *Evidence-based practice in nursing.* Springer Publishing Company.
- Chapter 3: Integrating Best Evidence Into Practice
- Chapter 8: How to Read and Assess for Quality of Research

Holly, C. (2019). *Practice-based scholarly inquiry and the DNP project.* Springer Publishing Company.

Holly, C., Salmond, S., & Saimbert, M. (Eds.). (2021). *Comprehensive systematic review for advanced practice nursing* (3rd ed.). Springer Publishing Company.

Oermann, M. (2023). *Writing for publication in nursing* (5th ed.). Springer Publishing Company.
- Chapter 6: Review and Evidence-Based Practice Articles

LESSON 5.2

FORMALIZING A PICO QUESTION

BACKGROUND

Think about the clinical practice problem that you have identified as well as the background information that you have collected. Now, you can begin formulating a PICO (population of interest/problem, intervention, comparison, and outcome) question to be answered. Your question will guide your literature search.

LEARNING OBJECTIVES

- Use the PICO format to develop a question.
- Organize PICO components into categories.
- Develop a list of synonyms for your literature search.

ACTIVITIES

Recall your problem, population of interest, potential intervention, and desired outcomes for your DNP Project. Formulate a draft PICO question.

P: Population of Interest/Problem = _____

I: Potential Intervention = _____

C: Comparison = _____

O: Outcome(s) = _____

PATIENT	INTERVENTION	COMPARISON	OUTCOME
What are the patient's most important characteristics? • Primary problem • Disease state • Coexisting condition **Describe your patient specifically:** • Sex • Age • Ethnicity • Socioeconomic factors	**What do you want to do for the patient?** • Order a diagnostic test • Prescribe a medication • Order a procedure	**What is the alternate intervention, if any?** • A different medication • No medication • A different test • A different procedure	**What are you hoping to achieve, measure, or change for the patient?** • Alleviate symptoms • Improve test results • Reduce adverse events • Improve function; could also seek an undesired result
ALWAYS include this piece in your search.	**ALMOST ALWAYS** include this piece in your search.	It is **LESS COMMON** to include this piece in a search.	**SOMETIMES** include this piece in your search.

To start, keep this simple. For the comparison, just say "usual care" or "current practice." If you are making a change in practice, the comparison is the current way things are currently being done. Your question may have more than one outcome. In this circumstance, you will still develop the question the same way.

It is important to avoid biasing your PICO question by including what you *want* to happen. Your PICO question should not be directional (e.g., improve, reduce). Keep in mind that we are not testing hypotheses. Example: Instead of stating, "Among patients with COPD (P), *does* a COPD action plan (I), compared to current practice (C), *improve* medication compliance," you could ask, "Among patients with COPD (P), *how does* a COPD action plan (I), compared to current practice (C), *impact* medication compliance."

When you see "PICOT," the letter *T* stands for "time." What period of time is involved? We recommend adding this later. Focus now on the skill of formulating a PICO question.

Example: "Among patients with hypertension (P), how does remote patient monitoring (I), compared to current practice (C), impact medication compliance (O)?"

P (Patient/population)	Patients with hypertension
I (Intervention/indicator)	Remote patient monitoring
C (Comparison/control)	Current practice (what is currently happening)
O (Outcome)	Medication compliance

☑ **Draft your PICO question:**

_____
_____
_____
_____
_____
_____

Now, identify the keywords of each PICO component and write them in each box. Then, try to think of different ways that word might appear in the literature. Make a list.

	KEYWORDS	SYNONYMS
P		
I		
C		
O		

Search databases are complex. We recommend that you seek assistance from your school's librarian to achieve the best results and utilize the appropriate Medical Subject Headings (MeSH).

☑ **Ensure that your question is a good question. Be prepared to answer these "FINER" questions (Christenbery, 2017; Holly, 2019):**

F: Is the question feasible?

I: Is the question interesting?

N: Is the question novel?

E: Is the question ethical?

R: Is the question relevant?

NEXT STEPS

- Consult with your faculty and mentor to review and approve your PICO question.
- Consult with a librarian in preparation for your database search.

REFERENCES AND RESOURCES

Christenbery, T. (Ed.). (2017). *Evidence-based practice in nursing.* Springer Publishing Company.
Holly, C. (2019). *Practice-based scholarly inquiry and the DNP Project* (2nd ed.). Springer Publishing Company.

RELATED TEXTBOOKS

Christenbery, T. (Ed.). (2017). *Evidence-based practice in nursing.* Springer Publishing Company.
  Chapter 6: EBP: Success of Practice Change Depends on the Question
Holly, C. (2019). *Practice-based scholarly inquiry and the DNP Project* (2nd ed.). Springer Publishing Company.
  Chapter 2: Practice-Based Scholarly Inquiry

LESSON 5.3

SELECTING APPROPRIATE DATABASES

BACKGROUND

After formulating your patient/problem, intervention, comparison, outcome (PICO) question, continue to identify synonyms for each component of your question. You will utilize the PICO question and associated synonyms when searching databases. A database is, in essence, a large electronic collection of information organized and cataloged for search efficiency. You must make a decision about which databases you utilize and determine those that will be most likely to house the information you seek.

Depending on the type of review you are doing, you will need to explore multiple databases. The PICO question and purpose of the review drive the type of review: (a) review of literature, (b) integrative review, or (c) systematic review (see table in Lesson 5.1).

LEARNING OBJECTIVES

- Review your PICO question, purpose of review, key terms, and potential synonyms.
- Read the descriptions of commonly used databases.
- Select databases that are most likely to yield information of interest.

ACTIVITIES

Complete the following prompts.

Your Problem Statement

_____

_____

_____

_____

Your PICO Question

P	
I	
C	
O	

What type(s) of review will you complete? Circle your answer.

- Formal review of literature
- Integrative review
- Systematic review

Commonly Used Databases

Review the descriptions and circle the databases you will utilize.

DATABASE	DESCRIPTION
CINAHL	The world's most comprehensive nursing and allied health research database. It provides indexing of the top nursing and allied health literature available, including nursing journals and publications from the National League for Nursing and the American Nurses Association. It also includes references and abstracts on nursing, biomedical, allied health, and consumer health literature; healthcare books; nursing dissertations; selected conference proceedings; standards of practice; educational software; audiovisuals; and evidence-based care sheets. Full text is provided for hundreds of journals, plus legal cases, clinical innovations, critical paths, drug records, research instruments, and clinical trials. **User tools:** Journal alerts, search-history alerts, saved search with personalized account, and compatible with most reference management software.
Cochrane Library	A collection of six databases that contain different types of high-quality, independent evidence to inform healthcare decision-making and a seventh database that provides information about Cochrane groups. All include full-text Cochrane systematic reviews. **User tools:** Journal alerts, search history alerts, saved search with personalized account, and compatible with most reference management software.
JBI	Database of systematic reviews that complement those found in the Cochrane Library. Includes a comprehensive range of resources, including more than 3,000 records across seven publication types, including literature reviews, recommended practices and procedures, information guideline sheets, comprehensive systematic reviews and protocols, consumer information sheets, and technical reports. **User tools:** Tools to create manuals and consumer information pamphlets and to adapt existing guidelines for local use. Tools to help users appraise individual papers using a checklist, conduct clinical audits, and develop systematic reviews of multiple papers.
MEDLINE	Widely recognized as the premier source for bibliographic and abstract coverage of biomedical literature. Provides information from the fields of medicine, nursing, and dentistry, as well as coverage in the areas of allied health, biological and physical sciences, humanities, and information science as they relate to medicine and healthcare, communication disorders, population biology, and reproductive biology. Contains more than 25 million citations from 5,200 biomedical journals published in the United States and other countries. Utilizes MeSH indexing with tree, tree hierarchy, subheadings, and explosion capabilities to search citations. **User tools:** Journal alerts, search-history alerts, saved search with personalized account, and compatible with most reference management software.

(continued)

DATABASE	DESCRIPTION
PsycINFO	Provides abstracts and citations from the scholarly literature in the behavioral sciences and mental health. Includes articles in psychology, medicine, psychiatry, education, social work, criminology, social science, business, and organizational behavior. This APA database includes material of relevance to psychologists and professionals in related fields, such as psychiatry, management, business, education, social science, neuroscience, law, medicine, and social work. Includes citations and summaries of peer-reviewed journal articles, book chapters, books, dissertations, and technical reports. Indexes more than 2,000 journals, 98% of which are peer-reviewed. **User tools:** Journal alerts, search-history alerts, saved search with personalized account, and compatible with most reference management software.
PubMed	Free search engine primarily accessing the MEDLINE database of references and abstracts on life sciences and biomedical topics. Comprises more than 29 million citations for biomedical literature from MEDLINE, life science journals, and online books. Citations may include links to full-text content from PubMed Central and publisher websites. The U.S. National Library of Medicine at the National Institutes of Health maintains the database. Most universities allow full-text holdings to be linked to citations. Indexed using MeSH. **User tools:** Journal alerts, search-history alerts, saved search with personalized My NCBI account, and compatible with most reference management software.
ScienceDirect (Elsevier)	Subscription-based access to a large database of scientific and medical research. Hosts more than 12 million pieces of content from 3,500 academic journals and 34,000 e-books. Journals are grouped into four main sections: physical sciences and engineering, life sciences, health sciences, and social sciences and humanities. **User tools:** Journal alerts, search-history alerts, saved search with personalized account, and compatible with most reference management software.
Scopus (Elsevier)	Citation and abstract database of peer-reviewed literature that can be used by researchers to determine the impact of specific authors, articles/documents, and journals. Contains more than 70 million records in the areas of science, technology, medicine, social sciences, arts, and humanities, with coverage strongest in the physical sciences (7,200+ titles) and health sciences (6,800+ titles), followed by the life sciences (4,300+ titles), and finally the social sciences and humanities (5,300+ titles). Titles are selected based on journal policies, content, journal standing, regularity of publication, and online availability. More than 25,000 titles (including open-access journals) from around the world are included. **User tools:** Journal alerts, search-history alerts, saved search with personalized account, and compatible with most reference management software, integrated with ORCID.

(continued)

DATABASE	DESCRIPTION
Web of Science (Clarivate Analytics)	Core Collection includes nine indexes containing information gathered from more than 20,000 scholarly journals, books, book series, reports, conferences, and more. The "cited reference" search is a main feature of Web of Science search capabilities. Provides complete bibliographic data, searchable author abstracts, and cited references Coverage is strongest in the sciences, followed by social sciences and then arts and humanities. **User tools:** Journal alerts, search-history alerts, saved search with personalized account, and compatible with most reference management software.
UpToDate	A point-of-care clinical evidence-based medicine database, providing coverage of more than 10,000 topics in 25 medical specialties. Integrates drug information (Lexi-Comp) and clinical images (Visual Dx). In addition to searching the entire resource or viewing topics by specialty, there are options to view the newest updates (What's New), practice-changing updates, drug information, and patient education information. **User tools:** Bookmarks, history, most viewed. Other features include standard medical calculators and a drug interactions analysis tool. Registered users can earn CME/CE/CPD credit.

APA, American Psychological Association; CE, continuing education; CINAHL, Cumulative Index to Nursing and Allied Health Literature; CME, continuing medical education; CPD, continuing professional development; EBP, evidence-based practice; JBI, Joanna Briggs Institute; MeSH, Medical Subject Headings; NCBI, National Center for Biotechnology Information.

You are encouraged to discuss your search strategy with a librarian. Understand that different databases use different terms and MeSH for different concepts. Databases may also utilize different symbols for truncation techniques. Completing this prework will make meeting with a librarian more productive.

NEXT STEPS

- Consult your school's librarian, in person or remotely.
- Prepare to keep track of your findings as you search.

RELATED TEXTBOOKS

Christenbery, T. (Ed.). (2017). *Evidence-based practice in nursing*. Springer Publishing Company.
    Chapter 3: Integrating the Best Evidence into Practice
Holly, C. (2019). *Practice-based scholarly inquiry and the DNP Project* (2nd ed.). Springer Publishing Company.
Oermann, M. (2023). *Writing for publication in nursing* (5th ed.). Springer Publishing Company.

LESSON 5.4

DOCUMENTING YOUR SEARCH, ANNOTATION, AND CITATION MANAGEMENT

BACKGROUND

As you review the literature, it is important to document your search strategy. Your documentation should be detailed enough so that your search could be re-created. Doing so adds credibility and transparency to your project, and as such, your search strategy will be documented in your manuscript. Depending on the requirements of your DNP Project, your search strategy may also be presented visually in a diagram.

You will read countless articles and therefore need to formulate a systematic strategy to annotate your work. Annotation refers to "close reading" or highlighting and making notes about what you are reading. Without annotation, you run the risk of not remembering what you read and risk citing information incorrectly. As you are reading, consider does this information answer your patient/problem, intervention, comparison, outcome (PICO) question? This chapter will review the pros and cons of manual annotation versus technology-based annotation.

The product of your literature search is evidence that must be cited. Most DNP programs use the American Psychological Association (APA, 2020) style manual. You are encouraged to catalog your evidence. Fortunately, technology is available to assist with annotation and citation management. These software options are vital when working with large amounts of information. Check with your school to see whether these software items are offered as part of your technology package.

LEARNING OBJECTIVES

- Utilize Boolean logic to search the literature.
- Document searches and the results of each search.
- Begin an organized process for annotation.
- Consider use of annotation and citation management software.

ACTIVITIES

Add your PICO question to your problem statement and keep it in front of you as you work. Begin to search in the databases you identified in Lesson 5.3.

Keywords Versus Subject Terms (CINAHL Headings or MeSH)

- Keywords are a good way to begin a search. Keyword searching is how you typically utilize search engines. Think of important words or phrases and type them in the search field. Remember, keyword searching may return many unrelated results.

- Generate keywords by describing important concepts in your own words. Make a list.
- Subject headings are assigned words or phrases used to label materials (similar to hashtags). Subject headings describe the content of each item in a database. Use these headings to find relevant items on the same topic. Searching by subject headings (descriptors) is the most precise way to search article databases. Searches using subject heading usually return relevant results.
- Whenever you find an article, identify the subject terms associated with it to use with subsequent searches.
- You may also search for subject terms within databases.

Connecting Your Terms

- Join similar concepts or alternate terms with "OR." Use **OR** to broaden your search by connecting two or more synonyms.
- Link different parts of your topic with "AND." Use **AND** to narrow your search: All of your search terms will be present in the retrieved records.
- Exclude concepts with "NOT." Use **NOT** to exclude term(s) from your search results.

Use Limiters Within Databases

- Depending on what you are looking for, you can use specific limiters to filter your results to make a search more precise.
- The most common limiter is articles from peer-reviewed journals. This will limit your results to scholarly journals that rely on experts in disciplines to review drafts of articles prior to publication.
- Other examples of limiters include evidenced based, clinical queries, age groups, sex, and publication type.

Narrow the Date Range

- Limit your date range to the past 3 to 5 years. This will give you the most up-to-date information for your DNP Project.

Personal Accounts

- Each database allows you to set up a personal account. With a personal account, you can save preferences, organize your research with folders, share your folders with others, view others' folders, save and retrieve your search history, create email alerts and/or rich site summary (RSS) feeds, and gain access to your saved research remotely.

Documentation

The National Institutes of Health (NIH, n.d.) recommends documenting the following search information:

- Complete, reproducible strategies
- Databases searched with date ranges (e.g., 2018–2023)
- Dates of each search
- Number of results from each search
- Number of duplicates removed
- Grey literature sources searched
- Other techniques:
  - Hand-searching
  - Bibliography/reference list review
  - Journal search
  - Author search

Keeping track of what progress you have made in your research is an important part of the research process. Consider the following questions. What databases have you used? What search terms and limiters have you used? Did you discover new keywords that you would like to try in future searches? What search techniques have been successful and unsuccessful? Knowing the answers to questions such as these can help prevent you from conducting duplicate research and overlooking valuable resources. I recommend that you maintain a database search log in a word-processing or spreadsheet program (Exhibit 5.1).

Exhibit 5.1 Sample Database Search Log

QUESTION	DATE	DATABASE NAME	SEARCH TERMS	SEARCH LIMITS	RESULTS
Does handwashing among healthcare workers reduce hospital-acquired infection?	April 12, 2023	MEDLINE (Ovid): 1946 to April 2, 2019	(handwashing OR hand hygiene OR hand disinfection) AND (cross-infection OR hospital-acquired infection)	English, Humans Last 5 years Adults Only Randomized Controlled Trials or Meta-Analysis	76 results

Gray Literature

Literature that is "semi-published" is not published and/or is not available through the usual bibliographic sources, such as databases or indexes, and is known as "grey literature." *Grey literature* takes many different forms but is essentially documentation that has not been formally published and has commonly not been peer-reviewed. Examples of grey literature include conference abstracts, presentations, and proceedings; regulatory data; unpublished trial data; government publications; reports (such as white papers, working papers, and internal documentation); dissertations/theses; patents; and policies and procedures. Sources may be oral, in print form, and increasingly, electronic formats.

Searching grey literature can be an overwhelming task. You should search those resources that make the most sense for your PICO question. At a minimum, consider searching conference abstracts, relevant stakeholder organizations, and online dissertation or thesis repositories. If your question involves medications and interventions, check clinical trial registries and pharmaceutical data. Sources for grey literature are consolidated in the table that follows.

GREY LITERATURE TYPES	GREY LITERATURE SOURCES
Abstracts and Conferences	- Conference Papers Index - Embase - F1000 Research Posters - NLM Gateway - Papers First - Scopus - Web of Science
Repositories or Reports	- Google Scholar - Grey Literature Report - The Joanna Briggs Institute - OAIster - Open DOAR - PROSPERO—International register of prospective systematic reviews - Virginia Henderson Repository
International Grey Literature	- Centre for Reviews and Dissemination (United Kingdom) - International Network of Agencies for Health Technology Assessment (INAHTA) - Institute for Scientific and Technical Information (INstitut de l'Information Scientifique et Technique—INSIST) of the French National Center for Scientific Research (CNRS; Centre national de la recherche scientifique) - International Clinical Trials Registry Platform (ICTRP) - Lenus (The Irish Health Repository) - National Academic Research and Collaborations Information System (NARCIS; the Netherlands) - Open Grey - RIAN (Pathways to Irish Research) - UK Clinical Research Network Study Portfolio - Virtual Health Library - World Health Organization (WHO)
Clinical Trials	- ClinicalTrials.gov - WHO - International Clinical Trials Registry Platform (ICTRP) - International Standard Randomised Controlled Trials Number (ISRCTN)
Regulatory Agencies	- Drugs@FDA - Devices@FDA - Health Canada Drug Product Database (DPD) - European Public Assessment Reports
Government	- NIH RePORTER (National Institutes of Health) - HSRProj (NLM; National Library of Medicine) - AHRQ (Grants On-Line Database) - Health Services and Sciences Research Resources (HSRR) - National Technology Information Service (NTIS)

Expert Commentary: Marilyn Oermann, PhD, RN, ANEF, FAAN

All literature searches should be done using a carefully developed and documented process. For many DNP Projects, conducting a well-planned literature review based on a search strategy (to ensure you have identified the relevant literature) is all that is needed. When conducting systematic, mixed method, scoping, umbrella, and other specific types of reviews, however, you need to use a methodological handbook or manual that outlines the step-by-step process to use. Two examples of these handbooks are the *Cochrane Handbook for Systematic Reviews of Interventions* (www.training.cochrane.org/handbook) and *JBI Manual for Evidence Synthesis* (https://jbi-global-wiki.refined.site/space/MANUAL).

You also need to follow guidelines for reporting the results of the literature search to ensure that it is complete and can be reproduced by others. One popular reporting guideline is the Preferred Reporting Items for Systematic Review and Meta-Analyses (PRISMA) (https://www.prisma-statement.org/?AspxAutoDetectCookieSupport=1). The PRISMA guideline is a 27-item checklist of information to include in the explanation of the literature search with a flowchart that documents the article selection process.

Your DNP Project is a good time to begin using reference management software, which allows you to save references found in a search and insert them into course papers and your DNP Project as well as manuscripts. Reference management software, such as EndNote and PaperPile, are proprietary and need to be purchased: check if your school provides free access to these. Other software programs, such as Zotero, are free.

NEXT STEPS

- Experiment and select your preferred annotation and citation management style.
- Complete your searches with assistance from faculty and librarians.

REFERENCES AND RESOURCES

Alberani, V., Pietrangeli, P. D. C., & Mazza, A. M. (1990). The use of grey literature in health sciences: A preliminary survey. *Bulletin of the Medical Library Association, 78*(4), 358.

American Psychological Association. (2020). *Publication manual of the American Psychological Association* (7th ed.). Author.

National Institutes of Health. (n.d.-a). *Documenting your work.* https://www.nihlibrary.nih.gov/services/systematic-reviews/documenting-your-work

National Institutes of Health. (n.d.-b). *Managing your search retrieval and analysis.* https://www.nihlibrary.nih.gov/services/systematic-reviews/documenting-your-work

National Institutes of Health. (n.d.-c). *Saving and updating the search.* https://www.nihlibrary.nih.gov/services/systematic-reviews/documenting-your-work

RELATED TEXTBOOK

Oermann, M. (2023). *Writing for publication in nursing* (5th ed.). Springer Publishing Company.

LESSON 5.5

OPTIONS FOR EVIDENCE APPRAISAL

BACKGROUND

After completing your literature search and reading and selecting the items to be included, it is time to critically appraise your findings. How do you know that an article contains "good" information? Was the study rigorous? Does the article help answer your clinical practice question? Your ultimate goal is to integrate the best evidence into practice (Christenbery, 2017).

The approach to evidence appraisal is determined by the purpose of the review and the type of evidence you are examining. For example, quantitative studies are appraised differently than qualitative studies. There is also a difference in appraisal of evidence that has been synthesized already (e.g., systematic review, clinical practice guideline) versus primary studies (e.g., randomized controlled trial, cohort study). In this lesson, the focus is appraisal of primary studies. Lesson 5.6 will review appraisal and reconciliation of clinical practice guidelines. To fully embrace appraising systematic reviews, training beyond this workbook is warranted.

Discuss evidence appraisal options with your faculty, as schools often adopt a particular method of evidence appraisal for DNP Projects. Although you may have learned about multiple evidence appraisal methods, you must be clear about your school's requirements. In this lesson, a broad overview of two commonly used evidence appraisal approaches is presented. Review the content, explore the online resources, and then talk to your faculty. You will need to select one strategy for your DNP Project and clearly articulate which strategy was used.

LEARNING OBJECTIVES

- Explore two commonly used approaches to rapid appraisal of primary studies.
- Select the strategy to be used in the DNP Project.

ACTIVITIES

So far, three types of literature reviews have been presented: formal, integrative, and systematic. The approach to literature appraisal largely depends on the type of review you are conducting.

DNP Projects will include a formal literature review as a component of the evidence-based practice process. Review the following evidence-based practice models, which offer approaches for rapid appraisal of evidence. Compare and contrast each approach.

- Evidence-Based Practice Process (Melnyk et al., 2010a, 2020b, 2010c):
    Critical Appraisal of the Evidence: Parts 1 to 3
- The Johns Hopkins Evidence-Based Practice Model:
    Appendix D: Evidence Level and Guide
    Appendix E: Research Evidence Appraisal Tool
    Appendix F: Non-research Evidence Appraisal Tool

SIMILARITIES	DIFFERENCES

NEXT STEPS

- Select the approach you will use for evidence appraisal. Discuss the approach with your faculty.
- After discussing the selected evidence appraisal approach with your faculty, begin your appraisal.

REFERENCES AND RESOURCES

American Association of Colleges of Nursing. (2015). *The doctor of nursing practice: Current issues and clarifying recommendations [White paper].* https://www.aacnnursing.org/Portals/42/News/White-Papers/DNP-Implementation-TF-Report-8-15.pdf

Christenbery, T. (Ed.). (2017). *Evidence-based practice in nursing.* Springer Publishing Company.

Dang, D., Dearholt, S., Bissett, K., Ascenzi, J., & Whalen, M. (2022). *Johns Hopkins evidence-based practice for nurses and healthcare professionals: Model and guidelines* (4th ed.). Sigma Theta Tau International.

Johns Hopkins Evidence-Based Practice Model. (2022). *JHEBP model and tools.* https://www.hopkinsmedicine.org/evidence-based-practice/models-tools.html

Melnyk, B. M., Fineout-Overholt, E., Stillwell, S. B., & Williamson, K. M. (2009). Igniting a spirit of inquiry: An essential foundation for EBP. *American Journal of Nursing, 109*(11), 49–52. http://forces4quality.org/af4q/download-document/3517/Resource-Evidence_Based_Practice__Step_by_Step__Igniting_a.28.pdf

Melnyk, B. M., Fineout-Overholt, E., Stillwell, S. B., & Williamson, K. M. (2010a). Critical appraisal of the evidence: Part 1. *American Journal of Nursing, 110*(7), 47–52. http://download.lww.com/wolterskluwer_vitalstream_com/PermaLink/NCNJ/A/NCNJ_541_516_2011_01_13_DFGD_5161_SDC516.pdf

Melnyk, B. M., Fineout-Overholt, E., Stillwell, S. B., & Williamson, K. M. (2010b). Critical appraisal of the evidence: Part 2. *American Journal of Nursing, 110*(9), 41–48. https://doi.org/10.1097/01.NAJ.0000388264.49427.f9

Melnyk, B. M., Fineout-Overholt, E., Stillwell, S. B., & Williamson, K. M. (2010c). Critical appraisal of the evidence: Part 3. *American Journal of Nursing, 110*(11), 43–51. https://doi.org/10.1097/01.NAJ.0000390523.99066.b5

RELATED TEXTBOOKS

Christenbery, T. (Ed.). (2017). *Evidence-based practice in nursing.* Springer Publishing Company.
  Chapter 3: Integrating Best Evidence Into Practice
  Chapter 6: EBP: Success of Practice Change Depends on the Question
  Chapter 8: How to Read and Assess for Quality of Research

Holly, C., Salmond, S., & Saimbert, M. (Eds.). (2021). *Comprehensive systematic review for advanced practice nursing* (3rd ed.). Springer Publishing Company.

LESSON 5.6

APPRAISAL, COMPARISON, AND RECONCILIATION OF CLINICAL PRACTICE GUIDELINES

BACKGROUND

Clinical practice guidelines are synthesized evidence. But are they the *best* evidence? White et al. (2021) examined 4,000 clinical practice guidelines and identified that only 14% were based on randomized controlled trials while 55% were based on expert opinion. You should therefore determine if the guidelines have been updated to reflect the most recent evidence. If guidelines reflect the most recent evidence and are well-developed, they could be considered good evidence for translation to practice. If you identify more than one clinical practice guideline on a given topic, the AGREE II tool can be used to compare and contrast the differences between guidelines.

LEARNING OBJECTIVES

- Build on the clinical practice guideline previously selected for the background of your DNP Project.
- Appraise individual clinical practice guideline(s) based on the Institute of Medicine (IOM) standards.
- Compare two clinical practice guidelines using the AGREE II tool.
- Reconcile clinical practice guidelines for translation to your DNP Project.

ACTIVITIES

1. Identify the clinical practice guideline you previously selected as part of your DNP Project background.

_____

2. Identify at least one additional clinical practice guideline on the same topic.

_____

3. Determine if there are any other guidelines available on the same topic. If so, list them here.

_____

_____

_____

☑ **Evaluate each clinical practice guideline. Do they meet the IOM standards?**

- Transparency
- Conflict of interest
- Diverse group composition
- Systematic review of literature
- Foundations for rating strength of recommendations
- Articulation of recommendations
- External review
- Updating

☑ **Select two clinical practice guidelines for comparison. Utilize the AGREE II tool to evaluate each guideline.**

SIMILARITIES	DIFFERENCES

☑ **Use the AGREE II tool to evaluate additional clinical practice guidelines, if necessary.**

Collectively, what are the recommendations?

What are the key differences?

Why do you think the discrepancies exist?

What are the key recommendations, regardless of guideline, that should be applied or translated to your practice situation?

Expert Commentary: Guideline Reconciliation in Hypertension: Irina Benenson, DNP, FNP-C, CEN

Appreciation for evidence-based clinical guidelines has grown during the past two decades. However, many guidelines provide conflicting recommendations on the same clinical issue, such as "hypertension" or "high blood pressure." It becomes challenging to adopt contradicting guidelines to the clinical practice or scholarly work. Inconsistent guidance commonly occurs when data are inconclusive and sparse and when guideline developers differ in their approach to evidence interpretation and synthesis.

For example, two sets of guidelines published in 2017 are aimed to address management of hypertension in older individuals (Qaseem et al., 2017; Whelton et al., 2017). Recommendations from the American College of Cardiology and American Heart Association (ACC/AHA) and the American

College of Physicians and American Academy of Family Physicians (ACP/AAFP) guidelines have many similarities. However, there is a substantial variation in guidance on blood pressure treatment goals (Benenson et al., 2019). The ACC/AHA authors support systolic blood pressure targets of less than 130 mmHg for older adults. On the other hand, the ACP/AAFP developers endorse a more conservative goal, below 150 mmHg, that is grounded in the total amount of evidence. What is the best guideline for your project, patient, or population?

This example illustrates how differences in the approach to data synthesis may impact treatment recommendations. No system is currently in place for reconciling differences. The solution here is for the DNP student, with faculty and preceptors, to carefully examine evidence, choosing recommendations that are applicable to the focus population and allowing options for decisions when the evidence is mixed or insufficient. That is, if the practice differences are unlikely to harm the quality of care. It is important to remember that decision-making regarding the care of the individual patient should always incorporate patients' personal preferences and perspectives.

When developing the DNP Project, the goal is to apply the best evidence that is aligned to the population of interest and desired outcomes.

NEXT STEPS

- Continue to discuss the development of your review of literature with faculty.
- Engage a librarian to assist with securing the best evidence.
- Remain organized as you review content using an annotation and citation management program.

REFERENCES AND RESOURCES

Benenson, I., Waldoron, F., & Bradshaw, M. (2019). Treating hypertension in older adults: Beyond the guidelines. *Journal of the American Association of Nurse Practitioners, 32*(3), 193–199. https://doi.org/10.1097/JXX.0000000000000220

Institute of Medicine. (2011). *Clinical guidelines we can trust.* https://www.nap.edu/read/13058/chapter/1

Qaseem, A., Wilt, T. J., Rich, R., Humphrey, L. L., Frost, J., & Forciea, M. A. (2017). Pharmacologic treatment of hypertension in adults aged 60 years or older to higher versus lower blood pressure targets: A clinical practice guideline from the American College of Physicians and the American Academy of Family Physicians. *Annals of Internal Medicine, 166*(6), 430–437. https://doi.org/10.7326/M16-1785

Whelton, P. K., Carey, R. M., Aronow, W. S., Casey, D. E., Jr., Collins, K. J., Dennison Himmelfarb, C., DePalma, S. M., Gidding, S., Jamerson, K. A., Jones, D. W., MacLaughlin, E. J., Muntner, P., Ovbiagele, B., Smith, S. C., Jr., Spencer, C. C., Stafford, R. S., Taler, S. J., Thomas, R., Williams, K., & Wright, J. T., Jr. (2017). 2017 ACC/AHA/AAPA/ABC/ACPM/AGS/APhA/ASH/ASPC/NMA/PCNA guideline for the prevention, detection, evaluation, and management of high blood pressure in adults: A report of the American College of Cardiology/American Heart Association Task Force on Clinical Practice Guidelines. *Journal of the American College of Cardiology (JACC), 70*(19), 1269–1324. https://doi.org/10.1016/j.jacc.2017.11.006

White, K. M., Dudley-Brown, S., & Terhaar, M. F. (Eds.). (2021). *Translation of evidence into nursing and healthcare* (3rd ed.). Springer Publishing Company.

RELATED TEXTBOOK

Christenbery, T. (Ed.). (2017). *Evidence-based practice in nursing.* Springer Publishing Company.

Chapter 9: Clinical Practice Guidelines

LESSON 5.7

CONSTRUCTING AN EVIDENCE TABLE

BACKGROUND

The purpose of an evidence table is to organize, outline, and present the findings of appraised literature in a succinct manner. Consult with your faculty to identify program requirements for what should be included in an evidence table. DNP programs may have established criteria for the number of studies to be included and format of the evidence table.

DNP students tend to be wordy when constructing an evidence table. Work to ensure that your wording is concise. The evidence table should present key, abbreviated information. As the evidence table catalogs your work, it should be included as part of your DNP Project proposal and final manuscript.

LEARNING OBJECTIVES

- Review evidence table exemplars.
- Organize your findings into an evidence table based on your school's DNP Project requirements.

ACTIVITIES

1. Review the article by Melnyk et al. (2010). https://www.nursingcenter.com/nursingcenter_redesign/media/EBP/AJNseries/Critical3.pdf
2. Create the outline for your table using their suggested headings:
    - First author, year
    - Conceptual framework
    - Design/method
    - Sample/setting
    - Major variables studied (and their definitions)
    - Measurement
    - Data analysis
    - Findings
    - Level of evidence
3. Populate the evidence table with your information into the designated columns.

NEXT STEPS

- Review your evidence table with your faculty and make revisions as needed.
- Prepare to write a synthesis of your findings in paragraph format.

REFERENCES AND RESOURCES

British Medical Journal. (2023). *Using BMJ best practice evidence tables and scores.* https://bestpractice.bmj.com/info/us/evidence-tables/

Melnyk, B. M., Fineout-Overholt, E., Stillwell, S. B., & Williamson, K. M. (2010). Critical appraisal of evidence: Part III. *American Journal of Nursing, 110*(11), 43–51. https://doi.org/10.1097/01.NAJ.0000390523.99066.b5

National Institute for Clinical Excellence. (2012). *Appendix K examples of evidence tables.* https://www.nice.org.uk/process/pmg4/chapter/appendix-k-examples-of-evidence-tables

RELATED TEXTBOOK

Christenbery, T. (Ed.). (2017). *Evidence-based practice in nursing.* Springer Publishing Company.

LESSON 5.8

SYNTHESIZING THE EVIDENCE

BACKGROUND

Now that you have collected and appraised the evidence for your DNP Project, you will synthesize your findings. Specifically, you will identify relationships, understand what is known, and describe any identified gaps (Oermann & Hayes, 2019). Synthesizing differs from summarizing in that synthesizing involves drawing conclusions, making connections, and showing relationships to your identified clinical problem rather than highlighting key points. As you are preparing to synthesize your evidence, consider the following questions. What does the evidence mean? How does the evidence relate to your identified clinical problem and population of interest? How will the evidence guide your project? The evidence table (Lesson 5.7) organizes your findings and will guide your synthesis

You should begin the literature review section of your manuscript by stating the question you are attempting to answer, followed by your search strategy. The strategy should be described in such a way that it could be reproduced and should include databases searched, key terms utilized, inclusion and exclusion criteria, and the number of articles identified. If you narrow the articles identified, describe how you approached that process. Details are important.

Next, you will present the findings. There are several ways to approach this step. Some utilize a chronological approach, discussing findings on a continuum. Others organize evidence into groups with each group addressing a component of the patient/problem, intervention, comparison, outcome, and time (PICOT) question. It is important to determine and discuss your approach with your faculty before you begin writing.

LEARNING OBJECTIVES

- Construct a paragraph describing your search strategy and findings.
- Outline an approach to a synthesis of findings.

ACTIVITIES

Use these prompts as an example of how to write an introductory paragraph for a review of literature.

The purpose of this _____ (type of review) is to answer the question (PICOT), "_____?" Selected databases for this review included (list databases) _____. Utilizing the key terms (list key terms), _____ a combination was entered _____ and tracked resulting in a total of (#) _____ results. The results were further narrowed by (inclusion/exclusion criteria) _____. After applying those limitations, a total of (#) _____ articles were selected for review. A synthesis of the findings is presented here.

Additional descriptors are required if you hand-searched the literature (e.g., review of reference lists). Inserting a diagram illustrating the search strategy and results is recommended. You may consider utilizing a PRISMA diagram to reflect your search strategy: https://prisma-statement.org/prismastatement/flowdiagram.aspx?AspxAutoDetectCookieSupport=1

Determine your evidence synthesis approach. Write an outline here.

_____

As you write any component of the DNP Project Proposal, we strongly recommend that you utilize anti-plagiarism software.

NEXT STEPS

- Enlist a classmate or colleague to read your paper.
- Ensure that a classmate or colleague can follow your search process and understand your findings.

REFERENCE AND RESOURCE

Oermann, M., & Hays, J. (2019). *Writing for publication in nursing* (4th ed.). Springer Publishing Company.

RELATED TEXTBOOK

Oermann, M. (2023). *Writing for publication in nursing* (5th ed.). Springer Publishing Company.
- Chapter 4: Reviewing the Literature
  - Exhibit 4.7: Analyzing Nursing Literature
  - Exhibit 4.12: Preventing Plagiarism

CHAPTER SUMMARY

A full description of your identified clinical problem is contained in the background and context section of your DNP Project proposal. Depending on your school requirements, the order of this chapter and Chapter 6, Framing the DNP Project—Taking Aim and Being SMART, may be interchangeable. This chapter presented you with invaluable knowledge to begin synthesizing and reporting your search strategy. Reflect on your work at this point:

What challenges are you experiencing?

_____
_____
_____
_____

What are two actions that you can take to resolve your challenges and move forward?

1.
2.

> Remember to maintain regular communication with your faculty, as this work is introductory and intended to give you a jump start. As a doctoral student, deeper engagement into evidence and literature is expected and required. Work hard.

NOTES

6

Assembling the DNP Project Team and Preparing to Lead Change

Editor: Tracy R. Vitale
Contributors: Molly Bradshaw, Mercedes Echevarria, and David Anthony Forrester

Lessons

Lesson 6.1 Historic Nursing Leadership to Frame Your Leadership Role

Lesson 6.2 You Are the Champion of Change

Lesson 6.3 Why Team Versus Committee?

Lesson 6.4 DNP Team Roles

Lesson 6.5 Creating Your DNP Team

Lesson 6.6 Considerations for Project Feasibility

Lesson 6.7 Articulating Desired Project Outcomes

Lesson 6.8 Writing a Purpose Statement

Lesson 6.9 DNP Project Theory

Lesson 6.10 Putting It All Together—An Outline

OBJECTIVES

In this chapter, you will build upon your problem statement. To recap, you have identified a problem and completed a review of literature to look for evidence-based solutions. Now, you will form a team to help you execute this work. It will be necessary to communicate clearly, ensure that your project is feasible (in your given time frame), and articulate the outcomes you want to impact. Your work should be based on theory. You should be able to describe all of this in a succinct way.

The goal of this chapter is to help you with assembling the DNP team, identifying a theory to base your work on, and drafting a problem statement. By the end of this chapter, you will be able to

- Build on the problem statement.
- Prepare to lead practice change.
- Assemble your DNP team.
- Identify theory to inform your DNP Project.
- Draft a purpose statement.

INTRODUCTION

To review, a DNP Project starts with a problem that impacts patients or populations, either directly or directly. What is the problem? What is the gap in practice? For this chapter, we will use the terms "problem" and "practice gap" interchangeably. We ask you to identify what the standard of care or current best practice is to address the problem or close this practice gap. It will become the basis of your intervention. Being able to clearly articulate this information will make you an effective champion of the practice change that is necessary.

Successful completion of a DNP Project requires the support of a team. There are some qualities and skills you need to understand as you build the team that will support you during this experience. Good leadership starts with good self-awareness, so remember to complete the suggested leadership evaluation tools in Chapter 1 of this text.

The American Association of Colleges of Nursing (AACN) recommends the group involved with the DNP Project at the academic level be called "DNP team" rather than "committee." The team is usually composed of the DNP student, a main faculty member, and at least one additional member. Often, a team includes a contact person at the organization or agency where the project will take place. Sometimes students have an influence in determining the members making up the DNP team. At other schools, the members are assigned. Likewise, the agency representative may not be optional. Before completing this chapter, it is a good idea to have your school requirements accessible as you work.

Remember the primary goal of the DNP team is to support you through this process. The DNP team assists the student in planning, data analysis, dissemination, and other critical project milestones. The expectation is that upon graduation, you will be skilled, experienced, and able to lead a change initiative independently. The final evaluation of the student is always the responsibility of the faculty (AACN, 2015). Again, refer to your school's requirements.

Based on our experience, we recommend that you keep the DNP team to as few members as possible. You can seek assistance and input from a multitude of sources. But it is not always necessary for the contributors to be an official part of the DNP team. The fast-paced realities of DNP Projects may not accommodate such a large team. Please ensure that you speak to your DNP chair first before officially seeking or inviting members to the team. The chair or faculty will help you decide whether the contributor should officially be on the team or not.

Students often feel conflicted about input they get from faculty teaching a course versus feedback from their DNP team. Who has the final say in green-lighting your project idea? Usually, the main faculty member assisting with your DNP Project is called the *DNP chair* or *DNP project advisor*. The DNP chair/project advisor may not be the faculty member teaching your project-related courses. In other words, you may be taking a class called "Project Planning" with a faculty member who is grading you on proposal development, but the actual approval of the proposal is made by the DNP chair/advisor and DNP team.

It is important to know how the academic organizational structure works. How will your DNP chair be selected/appointed? How are grievances handled?

The DNP student must also be a leader in the healthcare setting, not simply a manager (Forrester, 2016). What is the difference? Nursing leadership involves visionary, long-term thinking; behavior modeling; trust; and other qualities (Forrester, 2016). Nursing management takes a short-term and task-oriented view that maintains a status quo often by following rules and guidelines (Forrester, 2016). Nursing has a rich history of leadership. You will be joining its ranks. Take time to indulge in reading and learning about the plight of other nursing leaders. How does their work apply to the problem you are facing?

Next, the chapter includes a brief discussion of common change theories. Students will need to think about how theory may help with identification of project barriers and assist with facilitation of certain project components. Theories to inform project development may or may not be the same as those used to implement the project. More on this in our lessons.

Finally, we guide you through some exercises to help make sure you have thought carefully about the potential intervention(s), project feasibility, and outcomes. These points must be clarified before you write a purpose statement. The purpose statement builds on your problem statement.

You will need to arrange for a meeting and discussion with your project faculty when you have completed the work of this chapter. Do *not* move onto Chapter 7 without faculty approval of your DNP Project purpose statement, aim(s), and objectives.

MY GOALS FOR FRAMING THE DNP PROJECT ARE TO:

_____
_____
_____
_____
_____
_____
_____
_____
_____
_____
_____
_____
_____
_____
_____
_____
_____
_____

LESSON 6.1

HISTORIC NURSING LEADERSHIP TO FRAME YOUR LEADERSHIP ROLE

BACKGROUND

At the time I began studying for my DNP degree, I had been an RN for 15 years. I regret to report that I had never found the time to read Florence Nightingale's (1859) *Notes on Nursing*. Could I call myself an expert leader and know really nothing about the iconic nursing leaders?

During my doctoral education, I made a commitment to improve my knowledge of historical nursing leadership. They say history repeats itself. Could we appreciate historic nursing leadership to prepare us for new leadership roles in nursing? These leaders identified problems and found ways to make a change in practice and address the problems to improve outcomes for their patients. The process of problem-solving and concepts of leadership are not new. If they can lead, so can I, and so can you. —Dr. O'Neal

LEARNING OBJECTIVES

- Examine historic nursing leadership to inform future practice change.

ACTIVITIES

Identify five leaders of interest to you; here is a list of suggestions. Investigate and read about them. Next to each nursing leader, list the major health problem(s) these leaders challenged and the strategies they used to change nursing practice.

- Mother Mary Aikenhead (Irish; 1787–1858): Arguably the first visiting nurse in the world
- Dorothea Lynde Dix (American; 1802–1887): Widely known as a pioneer crusader for the mentally ill
- Florence Nightingale (British; 1820–1910): Acclaimed to be the founder of "modern nursing"
- Clara Barton (American; 1821–1912): Humanitarian and founder of the American Red Cross
- Edith Louisa Cavell (British; 1865–1915): World War I nurse heroine who faced a firing squad
- Lillian D. Wald (American; 1867–1940): Founded the Henry Street Settlement, which evolved into the Visiting Nurse Service of New York
- Clara Louise Maass (American; 1876–1901): Sacrificed her life in the fight against yellow fever
- Margaret Higgins Sanger (American; 1879–1966): Birth-control activist and sex educator who opened the first birth-control clinic in the United States and established Planned Parenthood

- Elizabeth Kenny (Australian; 1880–1952): Challenged conventional wisdom and promoted a controversial new treatment approach for poliomyelitis
- Mary Breckinridge (American; 1881–1965): Established the Frontier Nursing Service (FNS) to provide healthcare in the Appalachian Mountains of Eastern Kentucky
- Luther Christman (American; 1915–2011): Advocate for race and gender equality in nursing
- Mary Elizabeth Carnegie (American; 1916–2008): Fought for racial equality

SELECTED LEADER	PROBLEMS THEY FACED	STRATEGIES TO CHANGE PRACTICE

Are any of the problems or strategies relevant in the practice of nursing today?

Do their leadership strategies apply to your leadership of this project? List three useful points.

1.

2.

3.

Doctor of Nursing Practices and Nursing's Distinguished History of Leadership: D. A. Forrester

One of the key messages of the Institute of Medicine's (IOM) report on *The Future of Nursing: Leading Change, Advancing Health* (IOM, 2011) is that "Nurses should be full partners, with physicians, and other health professionals, in redesigning health care in the United States" (pp. 1–11). DNP-prepared nurses are expected to take on frontline leadership roles in evidence-based nursing practice, administration, education, research, and health policy making. DNP nurse leaders are needed to transform the healthcare system, and therefore advance the health of society. In the health policy arena, DNPs must recognize their role in leading policy making. They must be a visible and vocal presence on high-performing teams, advisory committees, commissions, and boards. Only then will DNPs and all nurses be full partners in advancing the nation's health systems and improving patient care (IOM, 2011).

DNPs must participate in leading the nursing profession and society into the future. Studying nursing leadership and nursing history through the stories of some of the nursing discipline's most prominent leaders fills an educational gap for many nursing students and nurses regarding nursing, nursing leadership, nursing history, and nursing's impact on society (Forrester, 2016). Historic nurse leaders exemplify courage, bravery, fearlessness, open-mindedness, and innovation.

Nursing's history is replete with the life stories of many great nurse leaders. Ours is a distinguished history of nursing leadership, activism, and impact. Over the centuries, nursing leaders have modeled vision, intelligence, resourcefulness, and political awareness. Nursing's leaders have demonstrated a continuing commitment to advancing the discipline and meeting the increasingly complex needs of society.

Although the fascinating life stories of so many historic nurse leaders were lived out long ago and far away, they are just as relevant today as when they occurred. These nurses' stories tell of the evolution of nursing and society over the centuries and around the world. Their stories facilitate an exploration of the very nature of leadership.

In the aggregate, nursing offers a compelling history not only of events and people within the context of their times but also of the contributions of so many visionary women who had the sheer courage, tenacity, and passion to move the nursing profession into the future—to the betterment of society around the world.

The domain of leaders is the future (Kouzes & Posner, 2017). DNP nurse leaders must lead nursing, health, healthcare, and society into a better future. "*Exemplary nursing leadership* is active, future-oriented, and produces change" (Forrester, 2016, p. 5). The life stories of nursing history's greatest leaders inspire DNP-prepared nurse leaders to become activist agents of change striving for a better future for nursing, health, healthcare, and society.

NEXT STEPS

- Continue to improve your knowledge of historic and current nursing leaders.
- Who are the current nursing leaders in your discipline? What do you know about them?

REFERENCES AND RESOURCES

Forrester, D. A. (2016). *Nursing's greatest leaders: A history of activism*. Springer Publishing Company.
Institute of Medicine. (2011). *The future of nursing: Leading change, advancing health*. National Academies Press.
Kouzes, J. M., & Posner, B. Z. (2017). *The leadership challenge* (6th ed.). Jossey-Bass.
Nightingale, F. (1859). *Notes on nursing: What it is and what it is not*. Harrison.

RELATED TEXTBOOK

Forrester, D. A. (2016). *Nursing's greatest leaders: A history of activism*. Springer Publishing Company.
   Part 6: Encouraging the Heart
   Part 7: The Future

LESSON 6.2

YOU ARE THE CHAMPION OF CHANGE

BACKGROUND

You have identified a problem. There is a practice gap. Something should be happening (best practice) but it is not. During the background investigation, and perhaps the formal review of literature, you should have explored what the standard of care is (current best practice). Based on what the literature says and the current context at the intended project site, do you see the implementation of this best practice as a fit for the organization to address the problem (practice gap)?

You need to make an argument for your intervention(s) of choice. What are you planning to do, and why would it work? What evidence exists to support your planned intervention? To lead this DNP Project, you must become the champion of change. The process starts by being able to clearly articulate your problem, the standards of care (best practices) related to that problem, and the reason that it is a fit for the organization or local context.

LEARNING OBJECTIVES

- Document the standard of care (current best practice) to address the problem/gap.
- List the possible interventions that may be used to address the identified problem/practice gap.

ACTIVITIES

Record your project's problem statement:

_____

_____

Based on your background, review of literature, and/or other evidence/sources, list the potential standard of care (best practice) you could implement to address the identified problem/practice gap. Cite the source.

STANDARD OF CARE (BEST PRACTICE)	FIT TO ORGANIZATION OR LOCAL CONTEXT
1.	
2.	

STANDARD OF CARE (BEST PRACTICE)	FIT TO ORGANIZATION OR LOCAL CONTEXT
3.	
4.	

Notes:

NEXT STEPS

- Discuss your list with your faculty.
- Continue to reflect on use of this best practice in the project context.

RELATED TEXTBOOK

White, K. M., Dudley-Brown, S., & Terhaar, M. F (Eds.). (2020). *Translation of evidence into nursing and healthcare* (3rd ed.). Springer Publishing Company.

Chapter 8: Methods for Translation

LESSON 6.3

WHY TEAM VERSUS COMMITTEE?

BACKGROUND

The American Association of Colleges of Nursing (AACN, 2015) recommended the term *committee* be replaced with the term *DNP Project team* to further differentiate the team overseeing the DNP Project from those assisting PhD students. Clear expectations are outlined by the AACN that the DNP Project team is made up of the student (or group of students), a doctorally prepared faculty member, and a practice-focused mentor and/or agency representative. Review your school requirements for minimum degree requirements. Additional personnel (e.g., experts, mentors) may also contribute to the project as needed in a formal or informal capacity (e.g., medical expert, librarian).

REMINDER: "Committee" is most commonly used for PhD candidates; "team" is the preferred term for DNP Projects (AACN, 2015).

It is important to recognize DNPs are expected to change practice through interprofessional collaboration. Domain 6 of *The Essentials* focuses on interprofessional partnerships with the goal of optimizing care, while also enhancing the experience and strengthening outcomes (AACN, 2021). This is realized through collaborative efforts required to work through the DNP Project. Depending on the nature of your project, you will work with various professionals such as advanced practice nurses, registered nurses, administrators, staff, and possibly interdisciplinary personnel, including physicians, pharmacists, politicians, and others. Everyone brings a different perspective and area of expertise to the table, yet all can provide insight to the project. A distinguishing feature of the DNP- versus MSN-prepared nurse is that the DNP nurse is not just a contributor, but a leader in this capacity.

LEARNING OBJECTIVES

- Outline the differences between committees and teams.
- Identify benefits of DNP teams over DNP committees.

ACTIVITIES

Consider how the roles and responsibilities of an interprofessional team for a community hospital vary from a rewards/recognition committee for a community hospital. Reflect on your experience with both teams and committees and identify the differences between the two.

_____
_____
_____

Write down at least two thoughts or questions you have for your faculty.

1. _____
2. _____

SUMMARY

Teams are different from committees. They include people who are all working toward a common goal and are much more inclusive. Start to hardwire your brain to refer to those who assist you with your project as your *DNP team members*.

NEXT STEPS

- During project planning, consider the nature of team dynamics.
- Be mindful and alert, looking for colleagues and faculty with interests like yours.

REFERENCES AND RESOURCES

American Association of Colleges of Nursing. (2015). *The doctor of nursing practice: Current issues and clarifying recommendations. [White paper].* https://www.aacnnursing.org/News-Information/Positions-White-Papers/DNP-Implementation-TF-Report-8-15.pdf

American Association of Colleges of Nursing. (2021). *The essentials: Core competencies for professional nursing education.* https://www.aacnnursing.org/Portals/0/PDFs/Publications/Essentials-2021.pdf

Committee. (2019a). *In Merriam-Webster's online dictionary.* https://www.merriam-webster.com/dictionary/committee

Team. (2019b). *In Merriam-Webster's online dictionary.* https://www.merriam-webster.com/dictionary/team

RELATED TEXTBOOK

Broome, M. E., & Marshall, E. S. (2021). *Transformational leadership in nursing* (3rd ed.). Springer Publishing Company.

Chapter 7: Building Cohesive and Effective Teams

LESSON 6.4

DNP TEAM ROLES

BACKGROUND

Define the roles on your DNP team. First, as a DNP student, you will experience a shift in your practice, leadership responsibilities, and expectations. As a doctoral student, you are held to a higher standard and expected to produce outcomes on a much higher level. The bar is justifiably raised and you are expected to meet, if not exceed, those expectations. Some students will have leadership experience. Others may be newly graduated from a BSN program. We are starting with your leadership role on the DNP team. Later, the skills that you learn can be translated to accomplish high-order practice.

Next, recalling the recommendations of the American Association of Colleges of Nursing (AACN, 2015), the DNP Project should have a team that includes a doctorally prepared faculty member who can not only serve as a mentor but also be responsible for the evaluation of the final DNP Project. Recognizing that at times there may be many hands in the pot, it is important to be able to differentiate everyone's roles and responsibilities, which may vary by school and program.

Traditionally, the role of course faculty is to provide you with the skill set related to the DNP *Essentials* as well as meet the expected competencies and sub-competencies. For example, course faculty may guide a student through a literature review or provide the logistics of writing the academic papers related to the project. If course faculty are different from your DNP Project team, it becomes even more important to recognize the relationships and determine their impact on the project.

DNP preceptors and organization representatives have roles in your DNP education and DNP Project. Under most circumstances, the DNP team will include the DNP preceptor or another representative of the partnering organization. This team member is the expert on practice and/or organizational context.

The role of the DNP preceptor includes being able to lead, teach, consult, coach, supervise, support research, manage, facilitate, and be a resource to the student. The role of the preceptor is not only to provide direct supervision in the DNP Project experience hours but also to guide your development in a clinical environment to promote both critical thinking and self-awareness. Regardless of your type of DNP program, your preceptors and organization required leaders will provide you with the support for you to develop the skills necessary to be a DNP.

Systems-based practice is the focus of Domain 7 (AACN, 2021). It is expected that you will not only be able to direct patient care but also that of the greater community and coordinate resources with the end goal of safe, quality, and equitable care (AACN, 2021). Your DNP skill set will include the ability to conceptualize care delivery models that are feasible within the current context of not only the organization but also the political, cultural, and economic state (AACN, 2006). AACN Domain 2 focuses on person-centered care. Although the preceptor may have a responsibility to the DNP student in the clinical setting, it is possible that skills learned may be of help as you navigate the DNP Project. In this lesson, we will guide you through a process to clarify roles and assemble your team.

LEARNING OBJECTIVES

- List key roles of DNP team members in the DNP Project.
- Gather information for creating the DNP team.

ACTIVITIES

Student Role

Refer to the DNP Project requirements at your school and answer the following questions:

1. What are your responsibilities as a student according to the requirements at your school?

2. Who is your primary DNP Project faculty member (i.e., your *chair*)? Or how is the primary faculty member chosen?

Primary Faculty (DNP Chair) Name:

Email/Phone Number:

3. How are additional DNP team members selected or chosen at your school? At what point in the curriculum is this decision made? As a discussion point with your faculty, you may pre-identify potential team members. Make a list and discuss with your primary faculty member.

Name:

Email/Phone Number:

Organization:

166 The DNP Project Workbook

Why this person would make a good DNP team member:

Name:

Email/Phone Number:

Organization:

Why this person would make a good DNP team member:

Name:

Email/Phone Number:

Organization:

Why this person would make a good DNP team member:

In reviewing this information, write down at least two thoughts or questions you have for your faculty.

1. _____

2. _____

The student is the leader of the DNP team and is supported by a primary faculty member and additional team member(s). Sometimes additional people will contribute to the project in formal or informal ways. You have the responsibility to lead the project from concept through implementation and dissemination.

ACTIVITIES

DNP Faculty, Chair, and Team Member Roles

Review any school content that outlines the responsibilities of the DNP faculty and DNP team members so that you know how they can support you through your project. Often, this information is in the DNP Project requirements for your school. List their primary roles/responsibilities as related to the DNP Project:

1.

2.

3.

4.

5.

In reviewing this information, write down at least two thoughts or questions you have for your faculty.

1. _____

2. _____

The faculty are available to support you in several ways. It is your responsibility as the team leader to ensure effective coordination with both your DNP Project course faculty and those associated with your specific DNP Project. Be prepared to use this knowledge when you create a communication plan for the development and writing of your DNP Project.

ACTIVITIES

DNP Preceptor Role

Next to each domain, list a potential skill that you can learn from the preceptor. Note how that skill contributes to your DNP Project.

DNP DOMAINS	SKILL TO LEARN/PROJECT CONTRIBUTIONS
I. Knowledge for Nursing Practice	
II. Person-Centered Care	
III. Population Health	
IV. Scholarship for Nursing Practice	
V. Quality and Safety	
VI. Interprofessional Partnerships	
VII. Systems-Based Practice	
VIII. Information and Healthcare Technologies	
IX. Professionalism	
X. Personal, Professional, and Leadership Development	

168 The DNP Project Workbook

The AACN (2015) indicates that it may be necessary for additional personnel to assist with the DNP Project throughout the project stages. However, having multiple team members may create a situation in which there are competing motives. At this point, we have explored the roles and responsibilities of the student, primary faculty, and DNP preceptor/organization representative. Do you need additional contributions to your project? There are pros and cons to having more people involved in the intricacies of the project.

ACTIVITIES

Additional Team Members—Pros Versus Cons

Consider the following examples in which additional team members may benefit or hinder the DNP Project process. Reflect on how you would best handle the situation and whether you would add the third person as a team member.

Example 1: A student is developing a quality improvement (QI) project focused on improving exclusive breastfeeding rates in the neonatal ICU. The student's team currently includes a faculty member who provides expertise in DNP Project writing/navigating institutional processes and a team member who provides clinical expertise as a doctorally prepared neonatal nurse practitioner. The student suggests adding a lactation consultant who is assigned to the neonatal ICU as a team member due to this person's expertise and likely investment in seeing this project succeed.

Example 2: A student is conducting a QI project to develop a code sepsis protocol for the ED of an acute care setting. Knowing there is a tremendous amount of literature and standards of care to review for both the background and the significance and formal review of the literature, the student is looking to include the librarian as a third team member.

Determine additional contributors who are potential team members; consider the pros and cons of adding them as official team members.

CONTRIBUTORS	PROS/CONS	DISCUSSION POINTS
1.		
2.		
3		
4.		

In reviewing this information, write down at least two thoughts or questions you have for your faculty.

1. _____

2. _____

SUMMARY

Various people may be able to provide guidance and assistance in the development and implementation of the DNP Project, but not all should be a part of the team. To move forward, it is important to understand the difference between potential contribution versus role responsibility. Consider the need for a formal role on the DNP team versus acknowledging their contributions in the final DNP Project. As a next step, discuss any potential team members with your DNP chair or primary faculty.

NEXT STEPS

- Continue to explore strategies to help you in the role of the leader of the DNP Project.
- Discuss your concerns with your faculty.

REFERENCES AND RESOURCES

American Association of Colleges of Nursing. (2006). *The essentials of doctoral education for advanced nursing practice.* https://www.aacnnursing.org/Portals/42/Publications/DNPEssentials.pdf

American Association of Colleges of Nursing. (2015). *The doctor of nursing practice: Current issues and clarifying recommendations [White paper].* https://www.aacnnursing.org/Portals/42/News/White-Papers/DNP-Implementation-TF-Report-8-15.pdf

American Association of Colleges of Nursing. (2021). *The essentials: Core competencies for professional nursing education.* https://www.aacnnursing.org/Portals/0/PDFs/Publications/Essentials-2021.pdf

Forrester, D. A. (2016). *Nursing's greatest leaders: A history of activism.* Springer Publishing Company.

RELATED TEXTBOOKS

Broome, M. E., & Marshall, E. S. (2021). *Transformational leadership in nursing* (3rd ed.). Springer Publishing Company.

   Chapter 6: Shaping Your Own Leadership Journey

   Chapter 7: Building Cohesive and Effective Teams

Forrester, D. A. (2016). *Nursing's greatest leaders: A history of activism.* Springer Publishing Company.

   Part 2: Modeling the Way

   Part 3: Inspiring a Shared Vision

   Part 4: Challenging the Process

LESSON 6.5

CREATING YOUR DNP TEAM

BACKGROUND

The DNP Project is led by the DNP student. The DNP student is supported by the DNP team. Most DNP teams are made up of the student (or group of students), a doctorally prepared faculty member (chair), and a practice-focused mentor, organizational leader, interdisciplinary leader related to the project, and so on (American Association of Colleges of Nursing [AACN], 2015). Additional personnel (e.g., experts, mentors) may also contribute to the project in a formal or informal capacity with varying levels of support.

LEARNING OBJECTIVES

- Review institutional requirements for DNP team members.
- Identify potential DNP team members.
- Select DNP team members.

ACTIVITIES

Identify at least one faculty member and one practice-focused expert who could potentially be members of your team. Include rationales for why you have selected specific personnel. You may return to this activity depending on the project progression rules at your school.

POTENTIAL ROLE	POTENTIAL TEAM MEMBERS	PROJECT CONTRIBUTION
1. DNP Project Chair		
2. Practice Expert		
3. Organization Representative		
4. Other Member		

SUMMARY

The team that you create will drive the project. Surrounding yourself with a team that can provide you with the guidance, support, and expertise you need will help you at the most critical times of the process. Discuss with your faculty/DNP chair the process for formally inviting members to the team.

REFERENCE AND RESOURCE

American Association of Colleges of Nursing. (2015). *The doctor of nursing practice: Current issues and clarifying recommendations. [White paper].* https://www.aacnnursing.org/Portals/42/News/White-Papers/DNP-Implementation-TF-Report-8-15.pdf

RELATED TEXTBOOK

Forrester, D. A. (2016). *Nursing's greatest leaders: A history of activism.* Springer Publishing Company.
    Part 2: Modeling the Way
    Part 3: Inspiring a Shared Vision
    Part 4: Challenging the Process
    Part 5: Enabling Others to Act

LESSON 6.6

CONSIDERATIONS FOR PROJECT FEASIBILITY

BACKGROUND

DNP students often have big dreams and big ideas. *This is wonderful!* However, we need a reality check. First, we want you to graduate. Throughout your journey you are collecting tools for your toolbox, and your DNP Project is your first attempt at building something from scratch to a finished project. Your project is meant to be a foundation of future scholarship (American Association of Colleges of Nursing [AACN], 2015). It must be designed in a way that it can be completed in a reasonable amount of time. Second, we consider the careful balance of an organization's desire to promptly address the problem with the reality of taking extended time to ensure the student gains appropriate skills for project planning, development, and management. Conversely, the sense of urgency to get a project done for school may or may not align with the needs of the organization or context of the project. The project feasibility must be discussed among faculty, mentors, and site personnel before you finalize your purpose statement, aim(s), and objectives.

LEARNING OBJECTIVES

- Outline considerations for project feasibility.
- Discuss these considerations with faculty and stakeholders.

ACTIVITIES

Reflect on the following:

1. What are your personal considerations for this project?
   - What do you hope to learn?
   - What do you want to change?
   - How does this build a platform for your future?
2. What are the DNP program considerations for this project?
   - Tentative graduation date:
   - Key school requirements:
3. What are the organizational/agency/context considerations for this project?
   - What is the tentative timeline for implementation of this project?
   - Are there any specific concerns?

Every project has challenges and potential barriers. You should complete an organizational, environmental, or community assessment to identify barriers and facilitators for successful implementation of your planned change. What barriers will you face? Ask yourself:

Q: Is the organization even ready for this change?

A: Consider using the Organizational Readiness to Change Assessment (ORCA) instrument (Helfrich et al., 2009) to assess this.

Q: What are some of the reasons standards of care (best practice) are not currently being utilized?

A: Consider using the BARRIERS Scale (Williams et al., 2015) to assess the following.

COMMONLY IDENTIFIED BARRIERS	COMMONLY IDENTIFIED FACILITATORS
Characteristics of intervention: - Cost - Time - Lack of precision - Not developed for users' need - Not designed to be self-sustaining Context of intervention: - Lack of organizational support - Competing demands - Lack of time/resources - Prevailing practice against the innovation Design of intervention: - Irrelevant to practice - Failure to evaluate cost, adoption, or sustainability - Low participation - Not aligned with organizational mission	[a]Facilitators largely depend on the organization Research/evidence is more likely to be used in environments where: - Staff development is frequent - There is low emotional exhaustion - Positive leadership What facilitators in your project context will help you? List them here based on your organizational assessment:

Source: Adapted from White, K. M., Dudley-Brown, S., & Terhaar, M. F. (Eds.). (2020). *Translation of evidence into nursing and healthcare* (3rd ed., p. 306). Springer Publishing Company.
[a]Not all inclusive.

What are your top three concerns/challenges for project feasibility? What can be done in the planning phases to address these concerns?

Concern 1:

Plan for minimizing/addressing this concern:

Concern 2:

_____

Plan for minimizing/addressing this concern:

_____

_____

Concern 3:

_____

Plan for minimizing/addressing this concern:

_____

_____

NEXT STEPS

- Revisit this lesson if needed.
- Revise your plans for your project to ensure feasibility.
- Consult with your DNP Project chair and/or DNP team.

REFERENCES AND RESOURCES

American Association of Colleges of Nursing. (2015). *The doctor of nursing practice: Current issues and clarifying recommendations. [White paper].* https://www.aacnnursing.org/Portals/42/News/White-Papers/DNP-Implementation-TF-Report-8-15.pdf

Helfrich, C. D., Li, Y. F., Sharp, N. D., & Sales, A. E. (2009). Organizational readiness to change assessment (ORCA): Development of an instrument based on the Promoting Action on Research in Health Services (PARIHS) framework. *Implementation Science: IS, 4,* 38. https://doi.org/10.1186/1748-5908-4-38

White, K. M., Dudley-Brown, S., & Terhaar, M. F (Eds.). (2020). *Translation of evidence into nursing and healthcare* (3rd ed.). Springer Publishing Company.

Williams, B., Brown, T., & Costello, S. (2015). A cross-cultural investigation into the dimensional structure and stability of the Barriers to Research and Utilization Scale (BARRIERS Scale). *BMC Research Notes, 8,* 601. https://doi.org/10.1186/s13104-015-1579-9

RELATED TEXTBOOKS

Christenbery, T (Ed.). (2018). *Evidence-based practice in nursing.* Springer Publishing Company.

    Chapter 15: EBP: A Culture of Organizational Empowerment

White, K. M., Dudley-Brown, S., & Terhaar, M. F (Eds.). (2020). *Translation of evidence into nursing and healthcare* (3rd ed.). Springer Publishing Company.

    Chapter 9: Project Planning and the Work of Translation

    Chapter 13: Interprofessional Collaboration and Practice for Translation

    Chapter 15: Best Practices in Translation: Challenges and Barriers in Translation

    Chapter 16: Legal and Ethical Issues in Translation

LESSON 6.7

ARTICULATING DESIRED PROJECT OUTCOMES

BACKGROUND

Those involved in a DNP Project have goals—something they want to see happen as a result of the project. The goals vary depending on perspective, but there is overlap and competing priorities. For example:

- Student goals: Graduation, leadership development, mastery of DNP competencies and sub-competencies outlined in *The Essentials*.
- Faculty goals: Meet curriculum and program requirements including competencies/sub-competencies, prepare students for new roles in nursing.
- Organizational goals: Implement change to bridge a practice gap, improve safety/quality.
- Patient goals: Improve health.

The point is for DNP students to appreciate the DNP Project more than what you want as a student. Part of leadership development is learning to lead and execute projects in a way that satisfies the needs of multiple stakeholders.

Goals can be translated into outcomes. Outcomes must be measurable to assess the impact of the change that was implemented. When developing the DNP Project, the goals may be diverse. However, the DNP Project outcomes must be tied back, either directly or indirectly, to the patient (American Association of Colleges of Nursing [AACN], 2015). Again, the purpose is to improve health outcomes.

LEARNING OBJECTIVES

- List the project goals based on stakeholder perspective.
- Translate the goals to specific project outcomes.
- Provide rationales for direct or indirect impact on health outcomes.

ACTIVITIES

1. Reflect on your problem statement and your overall work up to this point. List the goals of this project for the identified stakeholders. Then translate those goals into specific outcomes for your project. State the relationship (direct or indirect) the goal has to patient outcomes. Determine whether this outcome is measurable. When determining the outcomes you can ask yourself, "what is the change in practice/outcomes I want to see?"

Student goals:	Faculty goals:

Organizational goals:	Patient/population goals:

2. Target specific goals and translate them to potential project outcomes.

Outcome: Rationale: (How does it relate to the patient/population?)

Is this outcome measurable? Yes No Unsure

Outcome: Rationale: (How does it relate to patient/population?)

Is this outcome measurable? Yes No Unsure

Outcome: Rationale: (How does it relate to the patient/population?)

Is this outcome measurable? Yes No Unsure

3. Complete this process until you have listed all the outcomes for your project. The number of outcomes for each project may vary. Confirm that all stakeholders are satisfied with this plan.

NEXT STEPS

- Discuss the project outcomes with your DNP team.
- Ensure that the organization/agency supports your project goals and outcomes.

REFERENCE AND RESOURCE

American Association of Colleges of Nursing. (2015). *The doctor of nursing practice: Current issues and clarifying recommendations. [White paper]*. https://www.aacnnursing.org/Portals/42/News/White-Papers/DNP-Implementation-TF-Report-8-15.pdf

RELATED TEXTBOOKS

Hickey, J. V., & Giardino, E. R (Eds.). (2021). *Evaluation of health care quality for DNPs* (3rd ed.). Springer Publishing Company.
   Chapter 4: Evaluation and Outcomes

White, K. M., Dudley-Brown, S., & Terhaar, M. F (Eds.). (2020). *Translation of evidence into nursing and healthcare* (3rd ed.). Springer Publishing Company.
   Chapter 4: Translation of Evidence for Improving Clinical Outcomes

LESSON 6.8

WRITING A PURPOSE STATEMENT

BACKGROUND

The DNP Project begins with a problem. You were instructed on how to develop a problem statement. We now build on that work by drafting a purpose statement. The DNP Project moves in a linear direction to (a) identify a problem/practice gap, (b) explore solutions based on evidence and best practice, (c) determine goals and desired outcomes of those involved, and (d) state the purpose of the project. A purpose statement logically follows the problem statement. What does the DNP team want to accomplish? Think of it as your mission statement, the objective of the work. After completing this activity, we recommend that you keep your problem statement and purpose statement on an index card in front of you as you work. This helps keep you focused.

LEARNING OBJECTIVES

- Build on the problem statement.
- Add your purpose statement.

ACTIVITIES

Complete these prompts to formulate the purpose statement.

1. Restate your problem statement:
   _____
   _____
   _____

2. List your project outcomes (as defined by the project question and the input of the DNP team in Lesson 6.3):

    1.

    2.

    3.

3. Ask yourself, "If I conduct this project, will the problem/practice gap be addressed or resolved?" The purpose statement will need to include the following elements:

- The population who will be participating in the intervention
- The proposed method or intervention
- The setting the method will be implemented in
- The outcomes to be measured
- The time frame of the project

Examples: Effective Purpose Statements

"The purpose of this DNP Project is to implement an evidence-based protocol within a community health clinic for the use of the teach-back method to newly diagnosed diabetics to optimize self-care management over a 3-month period."

"The purpose of this DNP Project is to implement the COPD Action Plan offered by the American Lung Association to all patients diagnosed with COPD on the unit prior to hospital discharge to improve medication compliance, self-management, and prevent readmission over a period of 30 days."

4. Draft your purpose statement:
_____
_____
_____

The purpose statement will follow the problem statement. Although it would be nice for purpose statements to answer every who, what, when, where, and how question, it is not always feasible. Make sure you have included the pivotal transition phrases like:

"The purpose of this DNP Project is to . . ."

"The DNP team will . . ."

"The goal of the DNP Project is to . . ."

Write the problem statement followed by the final purpose statement here.

Problem statement:
_____
_____
_____

Purpose statement:
_____
_____
_____

NEXT STEPS

- Engage a classmate to review your work; revise as necessary.
- Discuss with your faculty, DNP chair/team, and site mentors.

REFERENCE AND RESOURCE

University of Arkansas. (n.d.). *Creating a purpose statement.* https://walton.uark.edu/business-communication-lab/Resources/downloads/Creating_a_Purpose_Statement.pdf

RELATED TEXTBOOKS

Bonnel, W., & Smith, K. (2018). *Proposal writing for clinical nursing and DNP projects* (3rd ed.). Springer Publishing Company.
Chapter 9: Guiding the Advanced Clinical Project: The Purpose of a Purpose Statement

LESSON 6.9

DNP PROJECT THEORY

BACKGROUND

Theories are often used to inform and guide project development. A single DNP Project may contain both a theory and an implementation framework. The purpose of the project theory is to explain, predict, or understand the problem, population of interest, or some element of the project. The theory helps the DNP student envision barriers and opportunities to facilitate obstacles. Then, the methodology of the project is designed based on an evidence-based practice implementation framework.

It is beyond the scope of this workbook to fully engage in discussing each possible theory. However, since the DNP Project is focused on change, we examine some change theories. This will be helpful in getting you started so that you can discuss it further with your DNP chair and DNP team.

LEARNING OBJECTIVES

- Determine the best options to guide your DNP Project.
- Sketch a conceptual framework for the project using the selected theory or framework.

ACTIVITIES

Research the following theories and consider how they apply to your DNP Project. Try to align the theory to your project context. Highlight your top two selections and discuss with faculty, the DNP chair, and DNP team.

- Lewin's Theory of Planned Change
- Roger's Diffusion of Innovations
- Lippitt's Phases of Change Theory
- Havelock's Stages of Planned Change
- Stages of Change Theory
- Social Cognitive Theory

Create a concept map that aligns the elements of the theory with your DNP Project.

NEXT STEPS

- Discuss your findings with your faculty, DNP chair, or DNP team.
- Revise your visual representation and use it to help you develop components of your project.

RELATED TEXTBOOKS

Christenbery, T (Ed.). (2018). *Evidence-based practice in nursing*. Springer Publishing Company.
  Chapter 7: Change Theories: The Key to Knowledge Translation

Utley, R., Henry, K., & Smith, L. (2018). *Frameworks for advanced nursing practice and research*. Springer Publishing Company.

White, K. M., Dudley-Brown, S., & Terhaar, M. F (Eds.). (2020). *Translation of evidence into nursing and healthcare* (3rd ed.). Springer Publishing Company.
  Chapter 2: The Science of Translation and Major Frameworks
  Chapter 3: Change Theories for Translation

LESSON 6.10

PUTTING IT ALL TOGETHER—AN OUTLINE

BACKGROUND

Before writing the DNP Project methodology, you need to prepare a document to kick off that process. Let's begin by drafting an outline of your work to date.

LEARNING OBJECTIVES

- Develop an outline for your project methodology.

ACTIVITIES

Complete this activity by filling in the information for your proposed project.

PROPOSED TITLE OF PROJECT (FEWER THAN 12 WORDS)	STUDENT NAME (YOUR NAME AND CREDENTIALS)	DNP TEAM MEMBERS AND ROLES

Partnering Organization	
Organization Contact	

PROBLEM STATEMENT
(WRITE YOUR PROBLEM STATEMENT)

PURPOSE STATEMENT
(WRITE YOUR PURPOSE STATEMENT)

DNP PROJECT THEORY
(DRAW THE ELEMENTS OF THE THEORY. THEN WRITE THE ELEMENTS OF THE DNP PROJECT AS IT RELATES)

RELATED TEXTBOOK

White, K. M., Dudley-Brown, S., & Terhaar, M. F (Eds.). (2020). *Translation of evidence into nursing and healthcare* (3rd ed.). Springer Publishing Company.

Chapter 9: Project Management for Translation

CHAPTER SUMMARY

You are now ready to begin developing the project methodology. Remember to communicate with your DNP chair and DNP team as you continue to work through this process. Reflect on your thoughts at this point:

List two "Aha" moments while developing your purpose statement, aim(s), and objectives:

1. _____

2. _____

What are your priorities as you move into the project methodology? Make a list.

1. _____
2. _____
3. _____
4. _____
5. _____

Keep working hard!

NOTES

7

Project Methodology: Develop, Implement, and Evaluate

Editor: Fontaine Sands
Contributors: Molly Bradshaw, Tracy R. Vitale, Debra Bingham, Nancy Owens, and Gina Purdue

Lessons

Lesson 7.1 Perspectives on DNP Project Methods

Lesson 7.2 Developing Aims and Specific, Measurable, Achievable, Relevant, Time-Bound Objectives

Lesson 7.3 Think Beyond Education

Lesson 7.4 Implementation Frameworks and DNP Project Design

Lesson 7.5 Intervention Population, Inclusion/Exclusion Criteria, and Recruitment

Lesson 7.6 Collaborative Institutional Training Initiative Training and Ethical Considerations

Lesson 7.7 Participation Consent

Lesson 7.8 Evaluation of Outcomes and Process

Lesson 7.9 Project Data and Plans for Data Analysis

Lesson 7.10 Timeline, Budget, and Resources

Lesson 7.11 Anticipated Findings

Lesson 7.12 Institutional Review Board: Application Considerations

OBJECTIVES

The DNP Project methodology is the road map of the project. It describes what will be done and how the outcomes and processes will be evaluated. In this chapter, you complete a series of lessons and activities to help you construct elements of the DNP Project methodology. The goal is to develop, implement, and evaluate evidence-based practice (EBP) solutions to the problem of interest. By the end of this chapter, you will be able to

- Construct a plan and draft components of DNP Project methodology.
- Determine the best approach for evaluation of outcomes and processes.
- Review criteria for DNP Project quality and rigor.

INTRODUCTION

Organizing the DNP Project methodology is a milestone in the DNP Project process. You have invested significant time and effort at this point to fully understand the problem in its local context. You have explored and appraised literature. You have met with your DNP team to determine what is needed to achieve the project outcomes. The methodology is simply a road map that explains in detail how this goal of improving health outcomes will be achieved. This chapter gets you started pulling the elements of the map together.

The chapter begins with a review of the American Association of Colleges of Nursing (AACN, 2015) recommendations for the DNP Project methodology. Before you begin the methodology development, ensure that you are in compliance with the rules and regulations at your school and partnering agency. What types of DNP Projects are allowed? Is there a preferred outline or way of writing the methodology? What are the requirements of the institutional review board (IRB)? At some schools, DNP Projects qualify for IRB exemption status. At others, the DNP Project must be reviewed by the IRB or undergo full review if vulnerable populations are involved. You must also know whether the agency has its own process for IRB or project approval. Gather all of that information before you begin work on this section.

Later, as you begin to formally write the methodology section of your paper, you may notice a shift in the tone of the writing compared to the beginning of the proposal. Writing the methodology is specific and prescriptive. It must be very clear and precise so that those reading your proposal can understand exactly what activities you plan to do to meet the proposed objectives and how you plan to measure/evaluate those objectives. It would be extremely helpful to reread examples of DNP Project methodologies from your school prior to starting your own. You may also consult a textbook dedicated to writing proposals (see the section "Related Textbooks").

In essence, developing a methodology is making a plan. As Dwight Eisenhower said, "Plans are nothing; planning is everything" (White et al., 2020, p. 199). It is important to consider and troubleshoot potential challenges. When this project is implemented, it is unlikely that everything will go 100% according to the plan. That is why it is important to create and evaluate both process objectives and health or system outcomes. Evaluating the process is essential to understanding what EBP interventions were successful and which ones need continued change.

A detailed plan will help you lead a team more effectively. You will not accomplish this project alone. Others will be involved. You have support from your DNP team. The method, or plan, will help your DNP project team, participants, and stakeholders have clear expectations and instructions. Let's begin.

REFERENCES AND RESOURCES

American Association of Colleges of Nursing. (2015). *The doctor of nursing practice: Current issues and clarifying recommendations*. [White paper]. https://www.aacnnursing.org/Portals/42/News/White-Papers/DNP-Implementation-TF-Report-8-15.pdf

White, K. M., Dudley-Brown, S., & Terhaar, M. F (Eds.). (2020). *Translation of evidence into nursing and healthcare* (3rd ed.). Springer Publishing Company.

MY GOALS FOR PROJECT METHODOLOGY ARE TO:

LESSON 7.1

PERSPECTIVES ON DNP PROJECT METHODS

BACKGROUND

The American Association of Colleges of Nursing (AACN) does not give specific recommendations for the methodology used in the DNP Project; it asserts that faculty should support innovation and evolve as the nature of practice evolves (AACN, 2015). Primarily, it emphasizes the importance of all DNP Projects having components of planning/development, implementation, and evaluation. Its position statement is intentionally broad. Key clarifying points include the following:

- Integrative and systematic review *alone* does not meet the requirements for the DNP Project because it lacks the components of implementation into practice (p. 4).
- Portfolios are tools to document and evaluate students rather than satisfy DNP Project requirements (p. 4).
- Group projects must demonstrate individual evaluation of each student (p. 4–5).
- Those who aspire to be nurse educators will need additional training beyond the DNP in the role of nursing education (p. 7).

The methodology of DNP Projects may borrow concepts from research; however, instead of generating new knowledge, the purpose of the DNP Project is to translate and implement evidence into clinical and/or system-level practice (AACN, 2015); in other words, to close the 17-year gap between the creation of the evidence and implementation into practice (Vincent et al., 2010).

The DNP Project is about leading evidence-based projects to create practice changes that result in the improvement of health outcomes for populations. Quality improvement (QI) has emerged as the dominant model for the DNP Project. QI utilizes a systematic process to identify a problem; analyze existing processes and data; then, design, implement, and evaluate evidence-based practice interventions to improve healthcare outcomes for specific populations. As a reminder, the Institute for Healthcare Improvement (IHI) offers a free training program on how to improve based on the *Model for Improvement*.

Depending on your DNP program's written project proposal outline, the methodology section may begin with identifying the DNP Project's goal and objectives. We will begin the methodology section with identifying the project's methodological design.

Methodology is related to the project design or methods used for the implementation, data collection, analysis, and evaluation of the project. As presented in Chapter 6, well-established project measures, such as process objectives and post-implementation outcomes, help establish the methodology design of the DNP project. For example, will the data collection methods used to measure the objectives be quantitative, qualitative, or both (mixed methods)? Will data be collected at one point in time (pre- and post-implementation) or at intervals over a period of time (monthly, quarterly, annually)? Does the project evaluate a comprehensive program or a single intervention?

The methodology section of your proposal will be an important part of your IRB application. IRB reviewers will be looking at the specifics in this section for determining the validity of your design to render the expected outcomes and potential risks to project participants. Please review the requirements of the IRB application as part of your planning process.

LEARNING OBJECTIVES

- Examine the required content for the methodology of the DNP Project.
- Gather perspectives and outline your approach.

ACTIVITIES

Review the DNP Project and IRB requirements for your school regarding methodology. Make a list of the required elements and key concepts.

Notes:

_____

_____

_____

☑ **Finally, consider evaluating the overall project as a whole. Consult with faculty and/or agency representatives to determine whether there is a standardized form used for the evaluation of QI projects.**

_____

Describe your plan to evaluate the project's overall process (i.e., participant and/or stakeholder satisfaction survey, demographic characteristics):

_____

_____

_____

_____

_____

_____

_____

NEXT STEPS

- Talk with your DNP chair and DNP team.
- Gather their perspective on the best method to use for your DNP Project.

REFERENCES AND RESOURCES

American Association of Colleges of Nursing. (2015). *The doctor of nursing practice: Current issues and clarifying recommendations. [White paper].* https://www.aacnnursing.org/Portals/42/News/White-Papers/DNP-Implementation-TF-Report-8-15.pdf

Institute for Healthcare Improvement. (2019). *How to improve.* http://www.ihi.org/resources/Pages/HowtoImprove/default.aspx

Melnyk, B. M., & Morrison-Beedy, D. (2018). *Intervention research and evidence-based quality improvement: Designing, conducting, analyzing, and funding* (2nd ed.). Springer Publishing Company.

RELATED TEXTBOOKS

Sylvia, M. L., & Tehaar, M. F. (2018). *Clinical analytics and data management for the DNP.* Springer Publishing Company.

White, K. M., Dudley-Brown, S., & Terhaar, M. F (Eds.). (2020). *Translation of evidence into nursing and healthcare* (3rd ed.). Springer Publishing Company.

Chapter 2: The Science of Translation and Major Frameworks
Chapter 8: Methods for Translation
Chapter 9: Project Management for Translation
Chapter 14: Information Technology: A Foundation for Translation

---

LESSON 7.2

DEVELOPING AIMS AND SPECIFIC, MEASURABLE, ACHIEVABLE, RELEVANT, TIME-BOUND OBJECTIVES

BACKGROUND

To review, the American Association of Colleges of Nursing (AACN, 2015) articulated several minimum expectations for DNP Projects:

- Focus on a change that impacts healthcare outcomes (directly or indirectly).
- Have a system or population focus.
- Demonstrate implementation in practice.
- Include an evaluation plan for process and outcomes.
- Include a plan for sustainability.
- Provide a foundation of future scholarship.

These standards can be used to guide the development of the aim(s) and objectives of the DNP Project. The purpose of the objectives is to precisely describe how the aim will be accomplished. In essence, the DNP Project will require development of an evidence-based intervention that is then implemented and evaluated. The project should be designed in a way that plans for sustainability, dissemination, and future scholarship of the students.

The aim of the DNP Project is to (project vision)
To achieve this aim, the DNP Project objectives are to

- Develop . . .
- Implement . . .
- Evaluate . . .
- With plans for:
  - Sustainability
  - Dissemination
  - Future scholarship

LEARNING OBJECTIVES

- Outline the DNP Project aim(s).
- Draft the DNP Project objectives using **S**pecific, **M**easurable, **A**chievable, **R**elevant, **T**ime-Bound (SMART) criteria.

ACTIVITIES

Apply the verbs *develop, implement*, and *evaluate* from the AACN (2015) criteria to the planning process for your DNP Project.

Project Aim:

We envision the aim of the project as one key sentence. It is meant to be visionary and all-encompassing. It could be considered a broader version of the purpose statement. Most likely, it will contain language about improving health outcomes for a population.

Write a Draft of the Project Aim

_____

_____

_____

For clarity and to streamline effort, we recommend using the verbs from the AACN (2015) recommendations to write the project objectives:

Objective—Develop: What intervention will you use?	List the steps necessary to accomplish this:
Objective—Implement: How will you implement the intervention?	List the steps necessary to accomplish this:
Objective—Evaluate: a. How will the outcomes be evaluated? b. How will the process be evaluated?	a. List the steps necessary to evaluate each outcome: b. List the steps necessary to evaluate the process:

✅ **Describe your thoughts on:**

Sustainability:

_____

_____

_____

Dissemination:

_____

_____

_____

Future scholarship:

_____

_____

The statement of the aim(s) and objectives should be brief but focused. Explicit detail is unnecessary; that is reserved for the project methodology (Key Differences, n.d.). In the next lesson, we will streamline each objective to ensure that SMART criteria are met. Depending on the requirements at your school, the focus and formatting of your DNP Project aim(s) and objectives may vary. The goal here is to prepare a draft, which will help you develop your project methodology. The project methodology is a more detailed description of how you will execute the work of the project.

Objectives speak to the action that must be taken to achieve the project aim. Verbs indicate action, and Bloom's taxonomy is a method of categorizing action verbs (Figure 7.1). Reflect on the verbs listed and gauge your project intervention. Your goal for the intervention is to *apply* evidence, *analyze* and *evaluate* outcomes, and *create* an improved healthcare outcome.

The SMART strategy for writing objectives is applied in multiple disciplines. The letters represent a required component of a good objective. Use the SMART strategy to ensure that your project objectives are well developed (SmartSheet, n.d.). Define each term that follows, then use this checklist to ask yourself, "Are your objectives SMART?":

S: Specific

M: Measurable

A: Achievable

R: Realistic

T: Time-bound

7 • Project Methodology: Develop, Implement, and Evaluate

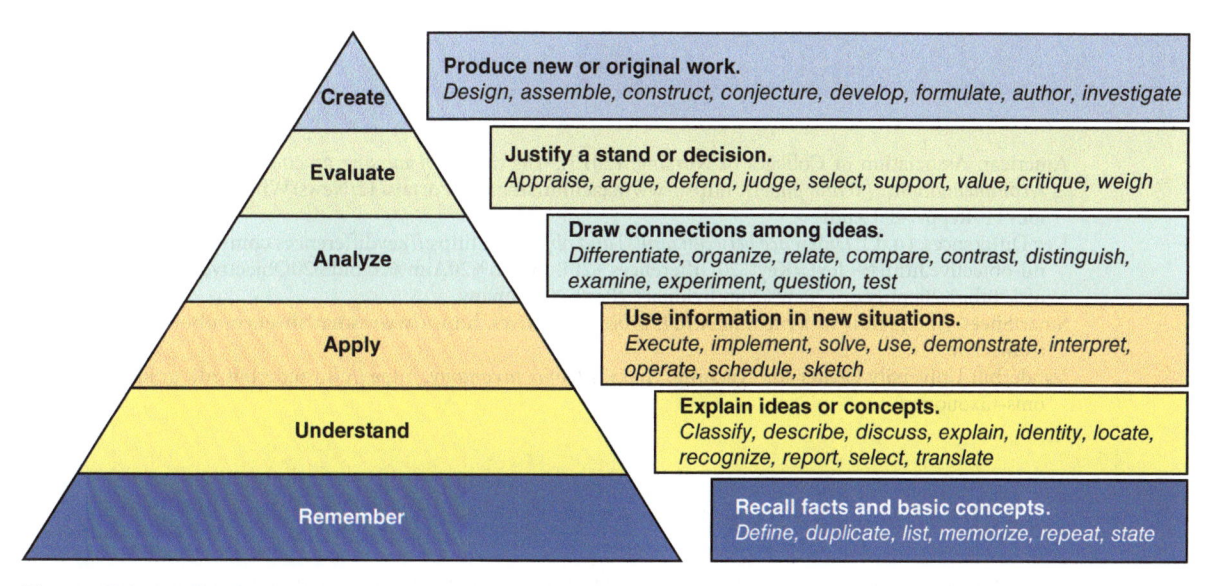

Create — Produce new or original work.
Design, assemble, construct, conjecture, develop, formulate, author, investigate

Evaluate — Justify a stand or decision.
Appraise, argue, defend, judge, select, support, value, critique, weigh

Analyze — Draw connections among ideas.
Differentiate, organize, relate, compare, contrast, distinguish, examine, experiment, question, test

Apply — Use information in new situations.
Execute, implement, solve, use, demonstrate, interpret, operate, schedule, sketch

Understand — Explain ideas or concepts.
Classify, describe, discuss, explain, identity, locate, recognize, report, select, translate

Remember — Recall facts and basic concepts.
Define, duplicate, list, memorize, repeat, state

Figure 7.1 Bloom's taxonomy.
Source: From Vanderbilt University Center for Teaching (n.d.). Bloom's taxonomy. Retrieved from https://cft.vanderbilt.edu/guides-sub-pages/blooms-taxonomy

ACTIVITIES

State your aim and objectives. Then review the objectives using the SMART checklist. Adapt the concept to meet your needs and school requirements.

Aim (Visionary statement of the project goal):
_____
_____
_____

Objective 1: Develop (State the key components.)
_____
_____

Objective 2: Implement (State the key components.)
_____
_____

Objective 3: Evaluate (State the key components.)
_____
_____

NEXT STEPS

- Review your final versions with your faculty, DNP chair, or DNP team.
- Do *not* proceed onto project methodology without approval of this content.

REFERENCES AND RESOURCES

American Association of Colleges of Nursing. (2015). *The doctor of nursing practice: Current issues and clarifying recommendations. [White paper].* https://www.aacnnursing.org/Portals/42/News/White-Papers/DNP-Implementation-TF-Report-8-15.pdf

Key Differences. (n.d.). *Difference between aim(s) and objectives.* https://keydifferences.com/difference-between-aim-and-objective.html#:~:text=Key%20Differences%20Between%20Aim%20and%20Objective&text=The%20aim%20of%20the%20entity,of%20an%20individual%20or%20company

SmartSheet. (n.d.). *How to write S.M.A.R.T. project objectives.* https://www.smartsheet.com/how-write-smart-project-objective

Vanderbilt University Center for Teaching. (n.d.). *Bloom's taxonomy.* https://cft.vanderbilt.edu/guides-sub-pages/blooms-taxonomy/

RELATED TEXTBOOK

White, K. M., Dudley-Brown, S., & Terhaar, M. F (Eds.). (2020). *Translation of evidence into nursing and healthcare* (3rd ed.). Springer Publishing Company.

Chapter 9: Project Management for Translation

LESSON 7.3

THINK BEYOND EDUCATION

BACKGROUND

We believe that nurses are born with a heart for teaching. There is something in our nursing DNA that tells us that education is always the right answer. Our instinct to teach others is rooted in good intentions. But the evidence says that education alone does not change behavior. In fact, when an educational intervention is delivered, it will only result in change 4% of the time (Institute of Medicine, 2011). To make a bigger impact on practice, we have to think beyond education. How can we get people to apply the information?

Almost every DNP Project involves delivery of information: an in-service training event, a simulated activity, or delivery of information to patients. We support the importance of this concept. However, best practices are necessary. You need to develop learning objectives and establish an evaluation plan for the educational session(s). We further recommend that there has to be some type of follow-up. How do you know the information is getting used and making an impact?

To make a bold statement, we believe the DNP Project must include an intervention that is more than just education alone. Measure something more than knowledge. Increasing awareness is great, but what is next? Did education improve confidence and/or competence (skill)? What tools are offered? What process or practice changes will be made? How will the outcomes be benchmarked over time?

LEARNING OBJECTIVES

- Determine what education is needed in your project.
- Plan the education event.
- Outline strategies to ensure the application and impact of knowledge.

ACTIVITIES

Answer the following questions:

- Will your DNP Project deliver information directly to patients or families?

Explain your vision:

- Will your DNP Project deliver information to healthcare workers?

Explain your vision:

When information is delivered directly to patients, here are some important considerations:

- Is the information based on evidence and is the source cited?
- Is the information written at the appropriate level of health literacy?
- Is the information culturally appropriate?
- How will the session take place? Individually? In a group?
- How long will each session last?
- What resources are needed?
- What are the intended learning objectives and how are the objectives evaluated?

☑ **The approach to education for healthcare workers may differ. When continuing-education credits are offered, there is generally a planning form required from the organization endorsing the content. Here are some important considerations:**

- Does the organization/agency you are working with have a form for educational events? (To view a sample educational planning form, refer to the editable forms supplement available at connect.springerpub.com/content/book/978-0-8261-7484-0/chapter/ch07.)
- Have you outlined the learning objectives?
- How will the knowledge be applied in practice?
- Does the evaluation of your educational session match up to the learning objectives?

☑ **After information and knowledge are delivered, regardless of the audience, how will the information be reinforced? Are there tools that you can offer to help remind the audience (e.g., handouts, pocket card, magnet, badge information card)?**

☑ **Now, think beyond education. What else needs to happen to ensure that there is a change in practice that impacts outcomes (directly or indirectly) for patients?**

NEXT STEPS

- Talk to your DNP team about interventions beyond education alone.
- Ensure that your DNP Project requires application of knowledge in practice.

REFERENCES AND RESOURCES

Bluestone, J., Johnson, P., Fullerton, J., Carr, C., Alderman, J., & BonTempo, J. (2013). Effective in-service training design and delivery: Evidence from an integrative literature review. *Human Resources for Health, 11*, 51. https://doi.org/10.1186/1478-4491-11-51

Institute of Medicine. (2011). *Clinical practice guidelines we can trust*. National Academies Press. https://www.nap.edu/read/13058/chapter/8#149

Medline Plus. (n.d.). *Choosing effective patient education materials*. https://medlineplus.gov/ency/patientinstructions/000455.htm

Strodtman, L. K. (1984). A decision-making process for planning patient education. *Patient Education and Counseling, 5*(4), 189–200. https://doi.org/10.1186/1478-4491-11-5110.1016/0738-3991(84)90179-4

White, K. M., Dudley-Brown, S., & Terhaar, M. F (Eds.). (2020). *Translation of evidence into nursing and healthcare* (3rd ed.). Springer Publishing Company.

RELATED TEXTBOOKS

Sylvia, M. L., & Tehaar, M. F. (2018). *Clinical analytics and data management for the DNP*. Springer Publishing Company.

White, K. M., Dudley-Brown, S., & Terhaar, M. F (Eds.). (2020). *Translation of evidence into nursing and healthcare* (3rd ed.). Springer Publishing Company.

Chapter 13: Education: An Enabler of Translation

LESSON 7.4

IMPLEMENTATION FRAMEWORKS AND DNP PROJECT DESIGN

BACKGROUND

In the previous lessons, you reviewed perspectives on DNP Project methods, looked at implementation science, and spent time thinking about interventions beyond education. Now, it is time to describe your project methodology by selecting an implementation framework. The implementation framework helps you design the project. This is an important step to consider because you want to use a framework that will fit with your aim.

LEARNING OBJECTIVES

- Explore implementation frameworks.
- Sketch the DNP Project methodology.

ACTIVITIES

Implementation frameworks will help you think through the elements of the DNP Project and operationalize the components. Explore each model and others if needed. Determine the best fit for your project.

- Institute for Healthcare Improvement (IHI) Model for Improvement (Plan-Do-Study-Act [PDSA])
- Iowa Model for Evidence-Based Practice (EBP)
- Knowledge-to-Action Model
- Agency for Healthcare Research and Quality (AHRQ) Knowledge Transfer Framework
- Ottawa Model of Research
- Reach, effectiveness, adoption, implementation, maintenance (RE-AIM) Model

Notes:

Selected framework: _____

Make a sketch of the elements of this framework.

Why is this framework a "fit" for your DNP Project methodology? List three reasons.

1.

2.

3.

☑ **Use your sketch created earlier. Next to the elements, describe the components of your DNP Project. You may need to revise your sketch after completing other lessons in this chapter.**

NEXT STEP

- Discuss your plan with your DNP team.

> **RELATED TEXTBOOKS**
>
> Bonnel, W., & Smith, K. (2018). *Proposal writing for clinical nursing and DNP Projects*. Springer Publishing Company.
>
> >   Chapter 10: Mapping It Out From Problem to Advanced Clinical Project Plan
> >
> >   Chapter 11: Writing the Methods Section: Organizing the Advanced Clinical Project
>
> Melnyk, B. M., & Morrison-Beedy, D. (2018). *Intervention research and evidence-based quality improvement: Designing, conducting, analyzing, and funding* (2nd ed.). Springer Publishing Company.
>
> >   Chapter 4: Using Theory to Guide Intervention Research
>
> Sylvia, M. L., & Tehaar, M. F. (2018). *Clinical analytics and data management for the DNP*. Springer Publishing Company.
>
> White, K. M., Dudley-Brown, S., & Terhaar, M. F (Eds.). (2020). *Translation of evidence into nursing and healthcare* (3rd ed.). Springer Publishing Company.
>
> >   Chapter 8: Methods for Translation
> >
> >   Chapter 9: Project Management for Translation

LESSON 7.5

INTERVENTION POPULATION, INCLUSION/ EXCLUSION CRITERIA, AND RECRUITMENT

BACKGROUND

The DNP Project is designed to impact patients and populations (American Association of Colleges of Nursing [AACN], 2015). To achieve this goal, the DNP Project intervention may or may not directly involve the targeted patient population. Often, the intervention population is not the same group. For example, if you are implementing a new protocol, the healthcare team will be the intervention population. In the methodology section, we need to identify the population participating in the intervention.

There may be reasons that you especially want to include or exclude project participants. You need to establish the rules for including or excluding people ahead of time. After the intervention population is identified, we will develop a recruitment strategy. How will the intervention population be made aware of your DNP Project? How, and by what means, will they be recruited to participate?

LEARNING OBJECTIVES

- Identify the intervention population.
- Outline inclusion/exclusion criteria of potential participants.
- Identify/develop plans for recruitment.

ACTIVITIES

What patient population is the DNP Project designed to impact?

_____

What population(s) will participate in the project intervention?

_____

Are there certain circumstances or rules by which you would include or exclude participants? List your inclusion/exclusion criteria.

INCLUSION	EXCLUSION

Recruitment Strategies

In our experience, most DNP Projects require a letter of introduction to the intervention population and a recruitment flier at a minimum. Please refer to the rules at your school and consult the institutional review board (IRB) as needed. A letter of introduction is a one-page, single-spaced letter that describes the context of the DNP Project. You should introduce yourself as a DNP student, state the full title of the project, and mention that this is a required component of your doctoral education. In the second paragraph, you should instruct the potential participant that participation is voluntary and there is no penalty for not participating. Next describe the intervention and the inclusion/exclusion criteria and outline what will happen. Describe the data-collection process and explain that the identity of the participant is protected. If the participant is being compensated for participation, describe the nature of the compensation. The letter should end by providing your contact information so that interested parties can follow up. The letter may also include the information of your DNP chair (faculty).

A recruitment flyer is simply a more concise, visual representation of the information included in the letter. It should contain the title of the DNP Project, provide a bulleted overview of the same elements described in the letter, and end with your contact information.

Both the letter and the recruitment flier can be circulated in a number of ways: personal communication, email, traditional mailing, and social media (if appropriate). There are often rules about proper ways to obtain contact information of participants and how this information is stored. Depending on your DNP Project approach, these may vary; consult with your DNP Project team and IRB.

Describe your strategies to spread the word about securing participants for your DNP Project:

_____

_____

_____

_____

Then, write a first draft of your recruitment letter.

> ☑ **To create the recruitment flier, use templates in Word, Google Forms, or other sources. Also, refer to the following resources.**
>
> - Free templates: www.designcap.com/create/recruitment.html
> - Community Tool Box: https://ctb.ku.edu/en/table-of-contents/participation/promoting-interest/posters-flyers/main

NEXT STEPS

- Consult with your DNP team.
- Revise your strategy as necessary.

REFERENCE AND RESOURCE

American Association of Colleges of Nursing. (2015). *The doctor of nursing practice: Current issues and clarifying recommendations. [White paper].* Retrieved from https://www.aacnnursing.org/Portals/42/News/White-Papers/DNP-Implementation-TF-Report-8-15.pdf

RELATED TEXTBOOKS

Melnyk, B. M., & Morrison-Beedy, D. (2018). *Intervention research and evidence-based quality improvement: Designing, conducting, analyzing, and funding* (2nd ed.). Springer Publishing Company.
  Chapter 14: Participant Recruitment and Retention
Sylvia, M. L., & Tehaar, M. F. (2018). *Clinical analytics and data management for the DNP.* Springer Publishing Company.

LESSON 7.6

COLLABORATIVE INSTITUTIONAL TRAINING INITIATIVE TRAINING AND ETHICAL CONSIDERATIONS

BACKGROUND

The Collaborative Institutional Training Initiative (CITI) Program is designed to ensure basic understanding of research-related ethics. Most schools require DNP students to complete this training, which is transferable to other universities. If the student remains involved in research and evidence-based practice beyond DNP graduation, it is necessary to periodically update one's training. Ask your DNP faculty about which modules are required for your school. To learn more, visit the CITI website (https://about.citiprogram.org/en/homepage).

In an effort to protect human subjects, there are some considerations to be made when including "vulnerable populations" in your project. This is specifically outlined in the U.S. Department of Health and Human Services (2018) Part 46 of Protection of Human Subjects. Examples of vulnerable populations include children, prisoners, pregnant women, victims of traumatic experiences, economically/educationally disadvantaged persons, and mentally disabled persons.

DNP Projects that include vulnerable populations often undergo full institutional review board (IRB) review regardless of the methodology of the project. Again, the purpose is to ensure humane treatment and protection for these populations. This type of information is included in the CITI Training.

When developing the DNP Project methodology, it is advisable to include a paragraph about relevant ethical concepts and the connection to the DNP Project. The American Nurses Association (n.d.) offers foundational content on ethical practice for all nurses (www.nursingworld.org/practice-policy/nursing-excellence/ethics).

LEARNING OBJECTIVES

- Ensure completion of required CITI Training.
- Identify vulnerable populations involved in the DNP Project.
- Articulate concepts of ethics applicable to the DNP Project.

ACTIVITIES

Then discuss CITI Training requirements with faculty and complete the required training. Ensure you get a copy of your completed CITI Training certificate, as the IRB may require it to be submitted with your application.

Questions for Consideration: Is there a vulnerable population involved in your DNP Project? If so, how will the risk to this group be mitigated in your DNP Project process?

☑ **Define the following ethical terms. Then write a paragraph about two terms and their relevance to your DNP Project. Use the National Institutes of Health (NIH) glossary to help you (www.niehs.nih.gov/research/resources/bioethics/glossary/index.cfm).**

Autonomy:

Justice:

Beneficence:

Nonmaleficence:

Fidelity:

Veracity:

Other term of your choosing:

Other term of your choosing:

Selected Ethical Term #1: _____

Write one paragraph on this term and its relationship to your DNP Project.

_____
_____
_____
_____
_____
_____
_____
_____
_____
_____

Selected Ethical Term #2: _____

Write one paragraph on this term and its relationship to your DNP Project.

_____
_____
_____

NEXT STEPS

- Discuss your work with your DNP team.
- Plan to mention ethical considerations in your DNP Project proposal.

REFERENCES AND RESOURCES

American Nurses Association. (n.d.). *Ethics & human rights*. https://www.nursingworld.org/practice-policy/nursing-excellence/ethics

CITI Training. (n.d.). *Research ethics and compliance training*. https://about.citiprogram.org/en/homepage

U.S. Department of Health and Human Services. (2018). *Part 46. Common Rule*. https://www.hhs.gov/ohrp/regulations-and-policy/regulations/45-cfr-46/index.html

RELATED TEXTBOOKS

Melnyk, B. M., & Morrison-Beedy, D. (2018). *Intervention research and evidence-based quality improvement: Designing, conducting, analyzing, and funding* (2nd ed.). Springer Publishing Company.

Chapter 7: Ethical Considerations in Designing Intervention Studies

Chapter 13: Navigating the IRB for Investigators

White, K. M., Dudley-Brown, S., & Terhaar, M. F (Eds.). (2020). *Translation of evidence into nursing and healthcare* (3rd ed.). Springer Publishing Company.

Chapter 16: Legal Issues in Translation

LESSON 7.7

PARTICIPATION CONSENT

BACKGROUND

Consent is a process, not just a form. Consent allows the potential participant to make an informed decision about whether to participate in a project/research study. This is "a fundamental mechanism to ensure respect for persons through provision of thoughtful consent for a voluntary act" (U.S. Department of Health and Human Services [USDHHS], 1993, para. 1). When you obtain informed consent, specific tasks and objectives must be met. These include having consent that provides information in a manner participants can understand. This includes all aspects of the project/study, including the project's purpose, the time commitment involved, what will occur during the project/study, alternatives, and any risks or benefits of participating (USDHHS, 1993).

Inclusion of participants, or their personal data, in the project requires some form of consent. Depending on the method, either a waiver of informed consent or informed consent is needed. It is necessary to consider the details of obtaining that consent. You need to describe the details and circumstances of how the consent will be obtained. The institutional review board (IRB) has standards and requirements. It will be necessary to familiarize yourself with any templates your project site or institution requires for consent. Consider that your institution may have templates for different types of consent depending on the nature of the project. Various consent types include written informed consent, parental permission form, paper or online survey/questionnaire consent, and waiver of informed consent. The type of consent that is required depends on the nature of the project you are conducting, the data you will be collecting, and the manner in which you collect the data.

LEARNING OBJECTIVES

- Describe the elements involved in informed consent.
- Determine the type of consent that may be required for your project.
- Identify special situations that may require additional consent considerations.

ACTIVITIES

Next to each prompt, answer the question in one to two sentences. Use the information as a foundation to construct your informed consent form for your DNP Project. Write as if you are speaking to the project participants. Use plain language.

Who is conducting the project? (Introduce yourself)	
What is the project about? (Problem and purpose statements)	

What is being done? (Overview of project intervention)	
What does the participant have to do? (Describe the participant role)	
Will there be compensation? (Describe the benefits of participating)	
Will there be consequences for not participating? (Describe what could happen by not participating. Could the person suffer harm?)	
How will confidentiality be maintained? (Explain the process of de-identification or securing of personal information)	
How much time will this take and over what period of time will the project occur? (Include intervention time and period of data collection)	
Who can the individual contact if they have questions? (IRB contact information for participant)	
Other:	

NEXT STEPS

- Discuss the plan with your DNP team.
- Retrieve your organization's requirements for when consent is required.
- Review available consent templates from your organization to review specific requirements.

REFERENCE AND RESOURCE

U.S. Department of Health and Human Services. (1993). *Office for Protection from Research Risks*. Informed consent tips. Tips on informed consent https://www.hhs.gov/ohrp/regulations-and-policy/guidance/informed-consent-tips/index.html

RELATED TEXTBOOK

Melnyk, B. M., & Morrison-Beedy, D. (2018). *Intervention research and evidence-based quality improvement: Designing, conducting, analyzing, and funding* (2nd ed.). Springer Publishing Company.
Chapter 7: Ethical Considerations in Designing Intervention Studies

LESSON 7.8

EVALUATION OF OUTCOMES AND PROCESS

BACKGROUND

The American Association of Colleges of Nursing (AACN) recommends that DNP Projects include evaluation of both outcomes and process (AACN, 2015). Reflect back on your project goal/aim and objectives. What outcomes were targeted? How will these outcomes be measured? DNP Project outcomes are often based on quality indicators, clinical measures, and other data. The process of making a practice change must also be evaluated.

Descriptive information, such as demographics, is helpful to articulate the composition of the population. It is also sometimes helpful to ask questions that confirm or deny findings in the literature. Do you need to formally complete a needs assessment? What was the opinion of stakeholders involved in the project? What went well? What could be improved?

The project evaluation plan will be individualized and should be planned with your DNP team. Since the DNP Project is a learning experience, you will benefit from interacting with multiple types of evaluations. You should incorporate different techniques.

EXPERT COMMENTARY

"I am often asked about the types of tools used to measure DNP Project outcomes. As faculty it's important to remember that I am teaching my students skills in data collection and analysis. To be fair and consistent, I recommend that each DNP Project contain one validated instrument, one self-developed instrument, and one data point that is benchmarked. That makes the work consistent between students and ensures that everyone is learning a consistent skill set. I further encourage at least 2-3 qualitative questions on the self-developed tool so that students gain experience in analysis of both types of data. I feel this approach best satisfies AACN's vision for competency-based education."

—Dr. Molly Bradshaw

LEARNING OBJECTIVES

- Explore validated instruments versus self-developed tools.
- Devise a plan for benchmarking outcomes data.
- Review strategies for survey development for the purpose of collecting feedback.

ACTIVITIES

Finding a data-collection instrument(s) that is right for your project is challenging. The instrument must measure the targeted outcome. The instrument must meet acceptable levels of *validity* and *reliability*. Some instruments may be used free of charge, whereas others may not. The DNP student may need permission from the developer to use the instrument. Developing a new, validated instrument is beyond the scope of a DNP Project. It is often more practical to use an instrument that has already been developed.

Expert Commentary: Tips for Finding Validated Instruments: Nancy Owens, DNP, APRN, FNP-C

Search the literature. Retrieve instruments that assess the practice-based problem in question. Databases may help you find out the name of an appropriate instrument, but it can still be difficult finding the instrument itself.

Assess each potential instrument. Identify those with established results and good indicators of validity and reliability. Has the instrument been extensively used by the scientific community?

Instrument sensitivity and specificity. Select an instrument that measures what you want to measure. For what purpose was this instrument developed? How was the instrument validated?

Contact the author or publisher for permission to use the instrument. You may be required to purchase the instrument. Consider the project or agency budget and time constraints.

Logistics. Consider the length of time required for completion of the instrument and complexity. Could your intervention population complete the instrument?

List your DNP Project objectives (process and outcome) and potential validated instruments to measure the appropriate objective. Discuss your findings with your DNP team.

Objective #1:

Potential Instruments:

Objective #2:

Potential Instruments:

Objective #3:

Potential Instruments:

Benchmarking Outcomes Data

In the quality-improvement process, benchmarking is a process of tracking an outcome over a period of time. This information can later be displayed as a run chart. For example, data may be collected from a patient chart by conducting a chart audit before the intervention (baseline data) and then at designated intervals after the intervention (post-implementation data). It may be necessary to develop a chart-audit tool or data-extraction form. If you are looking at multiple process objectives and outcomes, it can be helpful to have the information centrally organized.

Tips for Developing Chart-Audit Tools

1. **Determine the number of audits needed.** For most rapid-cycle quality improvement, 30 to 60 audits or 10% of the total population are rules of thumb (Agency for Healthcare Research and Quality, 2013). The number and approach should be discussed by the DNP team.
2. **Plan to collect data multiple times.** We recommend a minimum of three collection points for a DNP Project: baseline (pre-intervention) and two points post-intervention. Three data points can help determine trends. If available, trending data from the previous year(s) could be used to establish a baseline and/or comparisons.
3. **Privacy and data security.** *Never* take patient information from a chart without going through the proper channels. This process should not start until after the DNP Project proposal is fully approved and cleared by the given institutional review boards (IRBs; if applicable).
4. **Use guidelines, protocols, and standards of care.** These help to outline what information needs to be included in the tool.

☑ **Will your project benchmark contain clinical data points or performance measures? Develop a sketch of a chart-audit tool or data-extraction form. Present the sketch to your DNP team.**

☑ **Survey Development**

Surveys are developed for different purposes. DNP-prepared nurses require basic skills in survey development. The survey should collect information that is of value to the DNP team. Examples of feedback include demographics of the intervention population, validation of findings in the literature, documentation of needs, perspectives of stakeholders on current problems, and advice for improving the process for the next improvement cycle.

Resources for survey development: Survey Monkey. (2019). Survey 101. Retrieved from https://www.surveymonkey.com/mp/survey-guidelines

Vannette, D. (2010). 10 Tips for building effective surveys. Retrieved from https://www.qualtrics.com/blog/10-tips-for-building-effective-surveys

☑ **Consider the questions you will need to ask as part of your DNP Project. What will you need feedback on during this process? Draft the survey questions for review by your DNP team.**

Remember that when you are evaluating the overall DNP project process you will most likely need to develop your own tool or survey so that you can capture the data that are relevant to your project. The goal is to get feedback on what to improve during the next project or improvement cycle.

NEXT STEPS

- Review your evaluation plan with your DNP team.
- Ensure that both outcomes and processes are included.
- Revise your approach as necessary.

REFERENCES AND RESOURCES

American Academy of Family Physicians. (n.d.). *Eight steps to a chart audit for quality*. https://www.aafp.org/fpm/2008/0700/pa3.html

American Association of Colleges of Nursing. (2015). *The doctor of nursing practice: Current issues and clarifying recommendations. [White paper]*. https://www.aacnnursing.org/Portals/42/News/White-Papers/DNP-Implementation-TF-Report-8-15.pdf

Agency for Healthcare Research and Quality. (2013). *Practice facilitation handbook: Chapter 8, Collecting data with chart audits*. https://www.ahrq.gov/professionals/prevention-chronic-care/improve/system/pfhandbook/mod8.html

RELATED TEXTBOOK

Sylvia, M. L., & Tehaar, M. F. (2018). *Clinical analytics and data management for the DNP*. Springer Publishing Company.

LESSON 7.9

PROJECT DATA AND PLANS FOR DATA ANALYSIS

BACKGROUND

We would venture to say that when it comes to data and data analysis, there is a polar effect . . . you either love it, or it makes you cringe. We must recognize our limitations, and if you require help with part of the project, you should ask for assistance from data experts. Why must we even consider data analysis and statistics? Conducting data and statistical analyses allows us to interpret the results into useful, meaningful information. With the diversity of projects and designs, it is challenging to address all possible types of data analysis here, but we give you a jump start and explore common themes. Several important reminders:

- Make sure your measures match what you outlined in the aim(s) and objectives.
- Collect the exact same data at different points in time to benchmark appropriately. Analysis cannot be conducted if measurements are inconsistent.
- Don't forget to capitalize on collecting qualitative data via focus groups or open-ended responses on feedback surveys. There may be a unique perspective that quantitative measures fail to capture.

LEARNING OBJECTIVES

- Identify the dependent and independent variables of the project.
- Select the appropriate statistical test based on the type of data collected.
- Outline an initial data analysis plan.

ACTIVITIES

Simply put, the dependent variable is the outcome you are measuring.

Q: In this patient/problem, intervention, comparison, outcome (PICO) question, what is the dependent variable? "Among diabetics (P), what is the impact of a 5-minute counseling session (I) on fasting a.m. glucose (O) and A1c (O)?"

A: Fasting a.m. glucose AND A1c

The independent variable is the factor that you are planning to influence (intervention). The outcome that will be measured is the dependent variable. In this example, the independent variable is the 5-minute counseling session.

Write your PICO question:

_____

Based on your DNP Project, fill in the blanks:

INDEPENDENT VARIABLE (HINT: YOUR PLANNED INTERVENTION[S])	DEPENDENT VARIABLE (HINT: YOUR OUTCOMES THAT WILL BE MEASURED)

Before you select an appropriate statistical test, you must label the variable by category: nominal, ordinal, or scale (interval/ratio). Here are some definitions to help you:

TYPE OF VARIABLE	EXAMPLE
Nominal: Used to label or classify into groups or categories	Race, gender, hair color
Ordinal: Used to rank or order variables	Agree, neutral, disagree
Scale: Used when variables have a set standard of space	Temperature, blood pressure

All of these variables can often be analyzed using descriptive statistics (statistics used to describe a group of variables), including mean, median, mode, range, frequencies, percentages, and so on. You are trying to describe the variables. You are not really comparing them to anything at this point, just reporting them for what they are.

DNP Projects compare outcomes between two or more groups to draw conclusions (inferential statistics). To select the appropriate test, you must know the independent and dependent variables and know the type of variable (nominal, ordinal, scale). Common inferential statistics used in DNP Projects include a *t* test, paired *t* test, or analysis of variance (ANOVA). Here are some definitions to help you:

TEST	DEFINITION
t test	Used to test the difference between two groups
Paired *t* test	Used to test the difference between two groups at different points in time
ANOVA	Used to test the difference among three or more groups

Qualitative data are often collected in interviews, focus groups, or via open-ended questions on surveys. When the data are collected, they are reviewed, ideally by two reviewers. The reviewers each identify common themes. After they compare notes, they outline themes and derive the main point. The main point is sometimes translated into a synthesis statement—one single statement that captures the main point/idea. With this information in mind, outline your data analysis plan:

- Write your PICO question.
- Be clear on your independent and dependent variable(s).
- Pull each instrument used in the project.
- Determine whether it is quantitative or qualitative.
- Next to the quantitative measures, label the variable as nominal, ordinal, or scale.
- Mark your qualitative measures.

When this is complete, talk to your faculty about the best approach to use for data analysis.

NEXT STEPS

- Review your data analysis with your DNP team.
- Confirm that each of the data points you plan to collect is necessary and helps answer your clinical question.

RELATED TEXTBOOKS

Holly, C. (2019). *Scholarly inquiry and the DNP capstone*. Springer Publishing Company.
    Chapter 5: Qualitative Descriptive Research

Sylvia, M. L., & Tehaar, M. F. (2018). *Clinical analytics and data management for the DNP*. Springer Publishing Company.
    Chapter 1: Introduction to Clinical Data Management
    Chapter 2: Statistical Concepts and Power Analysis

LESSON 7.10

TIMELINE, BUDGET, AND RESOURCES

BACKGROUND

As a team leader, you are responsible for establishing the timeline and budget and identifying additional resources that may be required for your project. Appreciating the time and resources necessary for your project is just as important as the project itself. Establishing a timeline will allow you to keep yourself on track in an effort to meet the objectives of your project and ensure forward progress. Just as we have helped you bring a very broad, grandiose plan to a manageable size, we do the same in terms of setting a realistic timeline. Specific to the timeline, you may have an idea of when you expect milestones to be reached, but it is also important to consider the tasks that may be outside your control. This includes external and internal site institutional review board (IRB) approvals.

LEARNING OBJECTIVES

- Develop a project timeline.
- Organize a project budget and list necessary resources.

ACTIVITIES

Consider the time requirements of your academic program and how these align with your DNP Project. Establish a project timeline and consider the following milestones (at a minimum) and how long each will take:

TASK	START	DURATION
Project planning/proposal development		
Proposal approval (by DNP team)		
IRB submission/approval (site)		
IRB submission/approval (school)		
Implementation		
Data collection		

TASK	START	DURATION
Data analysis		
Writing results, discussion, implications		
Final presentation/dissemination		

Displays of your timeline should be easy to read and follow. You can develop a Gantt chart or create your own. Using the tools shown in Figures 7.2 and 7.3, create a timeline for the major milestones of your project.

Project Budget and Resources

As with any project, it is important to consider any costs associated with your DNP Project. Most times, the costs associated with a project are nominal, but you want to be mindful so you do not end up surprised by out-of-pocket expenses. In general, budgets consider both expenses and revenue related to the project. They also

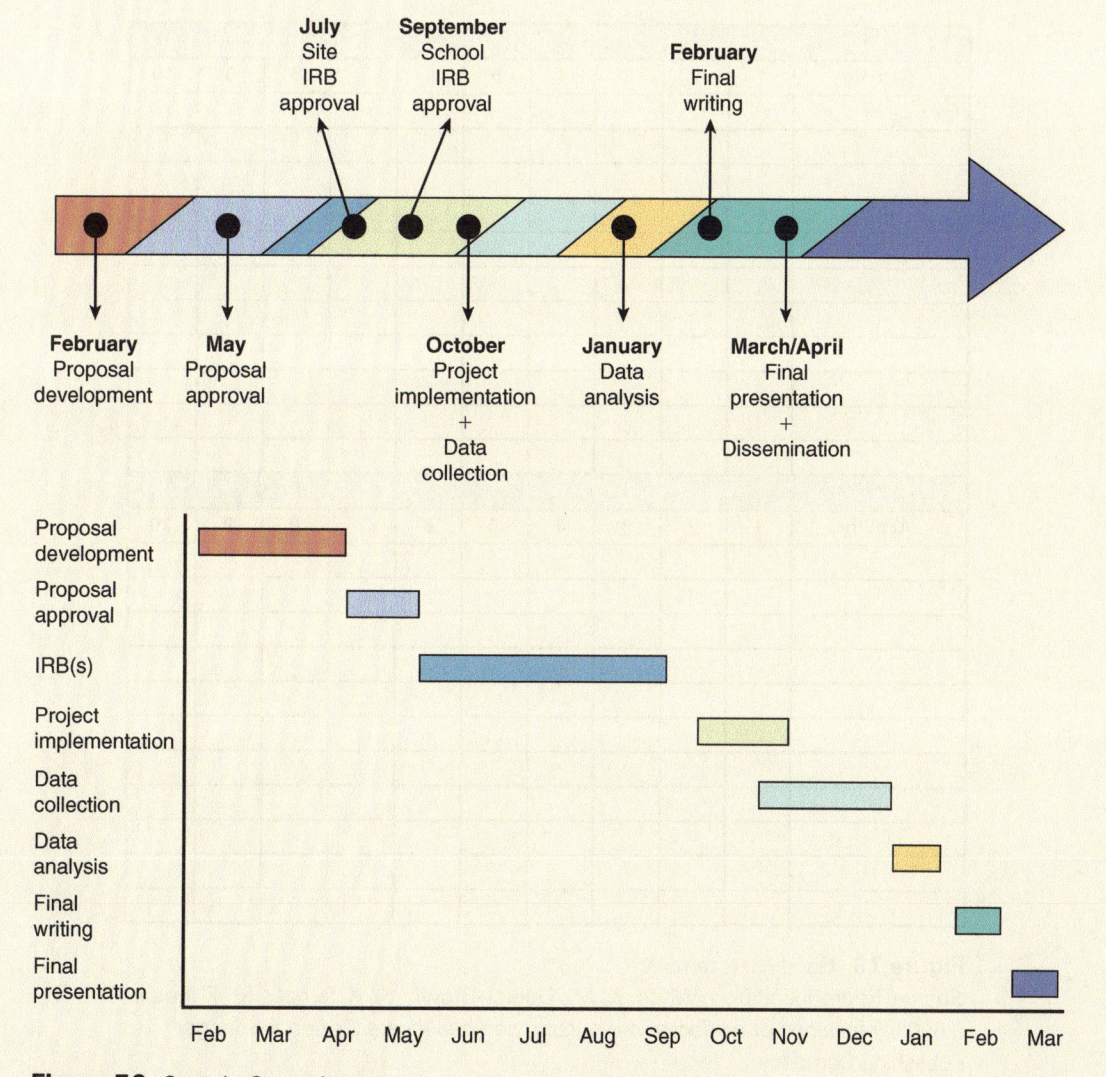

Figure 7.2 Sample Gantt chart.

include both direct (equipment/supplies) and indirect (day-to-day costs like electricity) costs. Consider the following types of expenses and resources that may be necessary specific to your project and establish an anticipated budget:

PROGRAM EXPENSE	PROJECTED COST	ACTUAL COST (ADD LATER)
Salaries/wages (admin support, practitioners, statistics consultant)		
Start-up costs (copies, charts, displays, etc.)		
Capital costs (hardware, equipment)		
Operational costs (heat/electricity)		
Other:		
Total Project Expenses	$	$

Figure 7.3 Gantt chart template.
Source: Reproduced from White, K. M., Dudley-Brown, S., & Terhaar, M. F. (Eds.). (2020). *Translation of evidence into nursing and healthcare* (3rd ed.). Springer Publishing Company.

NEXT STEPS

- Discuss your timeline and budget with your DNP team.
- Discuss the feasibility of the timeline in terms of providing enough time for each task.
- Consider how the timeline aligns with program requirements and your other academic responsibilities.
- Consider the required budget and resources. Are there opportunities for grant funding or donation of services?

REFERENCES AND RESOURCES

Smartsheet. (2019). *How to create a simple Gantt chart in any version of Excel*. https://www.smartsheet.com/blog/gantt-chart-excel

Teamgantt. (2019). *Free Google Sheets Gantt chart template*. https://www.teamgantt.com/google-sheets-gantt-chart-template

RELATED TEXTBOOK

White, K. M., Dudley-Brown, S., & Terhaar, M. F (Eds.). (2020). *Translation of evidence into nursing and healthcare* (3rd ed.). Springer Publishing Company.

Chapter 9: Project Management for Translation

LESSON 7.11

ANTICIPATED FINDINGS

BACKGROUND

What is it that you are trying to achieve by conducting your project? What are the data expected to show you? Consider the original aim of the project and the objectives you created in order to get there. Because you developed **S**pecific, **M**easurable, **A**chievable, **R**elevant, **T**ime-bound (SMART) objectives, you will be able to evaluate whether you successfully achieved them. In consideration of why you are doing your project, what do you anticipate your results to be? You need to consider the potential implications of your findings.

What are the potential facilitators and barriers to the project? How are you working to either remove them or use them to your advantage in the project?

LEARNING OBJECTIVES

- Describe anticipated project findings.
- Outline potential barriers to success.
- List potential strategies to mitigate barriers.

ACTIVITIES

Answer these reflective questions. Then translate your thoughts into a formal paragraph for your DNP Project proposal.

1. When you conduct this project, what do you think will happen? Will it be welcomed? Do you think the outcomes will be met? Explain.
2. What barriers to the successful implementation of your project exist? List them and then write a strategy to mitigate the barrier.

NEXT STEPS

- Translate your thoughts on anticipated findings and facilitators and barriers into two formal paragraphs for the DNP Project proposal.
- Discuss your concerns with the DNP team.

RELATED TEXTBOOK

Bonnel, W., & Smith, K. (2018). *Proposal writing for clinical nursing and DNP Projects.* Springer Publishing Company.

LESSON 7.12

INSTITUTIONAL REVIEW BOARD: APPLICATION CONSIDERATIONS

BACKGROUND

The institutional review board (IRB) is an entity designed to ensure humane and ethical conduct of research. The DNP Project is not research; however, the DNP Project must still be designed in a way that protects the project participants from harm. Human subjects research training is often required for any student, faculty, or essential staff looking to have a role in your DNP Project. Each school will have its own requirements for human subjects research training.

Although DNP Projects vary from school to school, a common debate revolves around the need for approval by an IRB. Quality improvement (QI) projects are geared toward improving the quality of programs, existing services, or a process flow. Depending on the nature of the project and the data being collected, it may result in the project being categorized as mandatory by the organization, thus not needing IRB approval, or required under the federal definition of human subject research, thus needing IRB approval. Regardless of how the organization classifies the project, most universities require students to obtain IRB approval.

7 • Project Methodology: Develop, Implement, and Evaluate   217

LEARNING OBJECTIVES

- Review the IRB requirements for your school.

ACTIVITIES

Review the IRB requirements for your school and partnering organization. Complete this planning form.

IRB Planning Checklist

Project Site Name	
Research Personnel Contact	
Required Process at Site	Site Approval Letter Only Yes ☐ No ☐ Nursing Research Council Yes ☐ No ☐ Research Council Yes ☐ No ☐ IRB Yes ☐ No ☐
Expected Time for Review	Nursing Research Council How often does it meet? _____ When are materials due? _____ How do I get on the agenda? _____ Research Council How often does it meet? _____ When are materials due? _____ How do I get on the agenda? _____ IRB How often does it meet? _____ When are materials due? _____ How do I get on the agenda? _____
Anticipated Type of Review	Exempt ☐ Expedited ☐ Full Review ☐
Required Supporting Documents	Human Subject Certification Yes ☐ No ☐ Informed Consent Yes ☐ No ☐ Recruitment Flier Yes ☐ No ☐ Data-Collection Tool(s) Yes ☐ No ☐ IRB Application Yes ☐ No ☐
Review Before Submission	Review of Application by Chair Yes ☐ No ☐ Consistency Throughout Yes ☐ No ☐ Written in Simple Terminology Yes ☐ No ☐ Attachments of Supporting Documentation Yes ☐ No ☐ Previous Approvals Yes ☐ No ☐

IRB, institutional review board.

Expert Commentary: Tips for the Method Section: Fontaine Sands, DrPH, MSN, RN, CIC—Nursing Professor and member of EKU IRB.

As a professor and an IRB reviewer, some of the common mistakes that I see students make in regard to the Methods section in the DNP Project proposal and IRB application is lack of detail. Both the DNP Project proposal and IRB application should discuss the steps of the project implementation in enough detail that non-nursing professionals can fully and clearly understand who the target population is, recruitment procedures, how the project interventions will be carried out, and how the project will be evaluated. To assist students in outlining the project in detail, I encourage them to begin by listing each objective (process and outcome), then list each activity or implementation steps the project leader will do and what the participants will do for each associated project objective. A timeline can then be created to help display the interventions and expected outcomes. This should help ensure no implementation activity is missed. A Gantt chart can be created listing the activities the project leader will do, and the participant activities need to be the focus in the IRB application methodology section.

NEXT STEPS

- Discuss your IRB status with your DNP team.
- Plan for timely submission of your required documentation.

REFERENCES AND RESOURCES

American Nurses Association. (n.d.). *Ethics & human rights.* https://www.nursingworld.org/practice-policy/nursing-excellence/ethics

CITI Training. (n.d.). *Research ethics and compliance training.* https://about.citiprogram.org/en/homepage

U.S. Department of Health and Human Services. (2018). *Part 46. Common Rule.* https://www.hhs.gov/ohrp/regulations-and-policy/regulations/45-cfr-46/index.html

CHAPTER SUMMARY

To review, the methodology of the project describes the processes followed by the intended intervention and includes an evaluation plan. This chapter engaged you in the prework and planning required to develop a successful DNP Project. Your DNP team should be involved in this process. Use this methodology outline as you prepare your DNP Project proposal.

Methodology Outline

DNP PROJECT AIM

OBJECTIVE	MEASUREMENT OF OBJECTIVE

Sketch of Implementation Framework:

Intervention Population:	
Recruitment Plan:	
Ethics: • CITI Complete • Ethical Review • IRB Required?	
Description of Intervention	

TOOL	DESCRIPTION	PERMISSION TO USE?
Self-Developed Tool(s)	Statistical analysis to be used?	
Validated Instrument(s)	Statistical analysis to be used?	
Benchmark(s)	Statistical analysis to be used?	

Plan for data storage?

Timeline:

Budget:

Plans for sustainability:

Anticipated findings:

8

Strategies to Organize, Disseminate, and Sustain DNP Project Findings

Editor: Tracy R. Vitale
Contributors: Molly Bradshaw, Thomas Christenbery, and David G. Campbell-O'Dell

Lessons

Lesson 8.1 Project Management

Lesson 8.2 Writing the Results and Discussion Sections

Lesson 8.3 Writing About Impact and Implications

Lesson 8.4 Completing the Final Academic Paper

Lesson 8.5 Skills for Oral Presentations

Lesson 8.6 Strategies for Creating Scholarly Posters

Lesson 8.7 DNP Project Repositories

Lesson 8.8 Social Media and Alternative Dissemination

OBJECTIVES

Organizations play a key role in successful DNP management. After the implementation of the DNP Project, the student must analyze data, interpret the findings, and finalize a strategy for sustainability. Upon completion, students are required to present the final academic products of the DNP Project, which include a paper, presentation, and poster. Beyond the academic setting, it is also important to relay the project findings to site personnel, colleagues, and the community. Storing and sharing DNP Projects in electronic repositories is considered best practice. In this chapter, students will examine skills for project management, composing final academic products, and plan dissemination of information in appropriate formats to others. By the end of this chapter, you will be able to

- Consider best practices of project management.
- Finalize plans for sustainability after data collection.
- Develop a plan to finish the academic products.
- Utilize multiple formats for dissemination of project findings.

INTRODUCTION

The proposed DNP Project must be approved by the DNP team, the institutional review board (IRB), and other appropriate entities before project implementation begins. As the project gets underway, you must stay organized and utilize your leadership skills for successful project management.

Detailed data-management strategies and clinical analytics are beyond the scope of this workbook. However, we advise you to consult with your faculty and other experts with skill sets to help you set up code books, use data-analysis software, and accurately interpret your findings. Several textbooks are also available for support.

You will need to consider the impact of the intervention on identified outcomes for the targeted population. What contribution did your project make to the organization, education, practice, policy, and health systems? You will make final plans for project sustainability. Likewise, you will examine the process itself and make recommendations about what could be improved.

All this information must be communicated. In the academic setting you will most likely be asked to present a final academic paper with an oral presentation. The paper generally builds on the DNP Project proposal. The proposal is changed to past tense. Instead of saying what will happen, the tone shifts to what was done. Then additional sections are added beyond the methodology such as results, discussion, and implications. The oral presentation is just an alternate format of the academic paper content. DNP students should have skills to present information in multiple ways. Again, we support the concept of the 3P's of academic products: paper, presentation, and scholarly poster (White et al., 2020).

Remember to check the requirements at your school. We discuss the differences between digital repositories and peer-reviewed publications. Social media considerations are outlined. Presenting information to contributors, the community, and patient populations may require a different approach, and you may need to revise your original plans depending on your project findings. Let's begin.

REFERENCES AND RESOURCES

Sylvia, M. L., & Terhaar, M. F. (2018). *Clinical analytics and data management for the DNP* (3rd ed.). Springer Publishing Company.

White, K. M., Dudley-Brown, S., & Terhaar, M. F (Eds.). (2020). *Translation of evidence into nursing and healthcare* (3rd ed.). Springer Publishing Company.

MY GOALS FOR STRATEGIES TO ORGANIZE, DISSEMINATE, AND SUSTAIN DNP PROJECT FINDINGS ARE TO:

LESSON 8.1

PROJECT MANAGEMENT

BACKGROUND

In addition to leadership skills, the DNP student must demonstrate an ability to manage the implementation of the DNP Project. Effective project management often translates to project success and includes emotional intelligence.

LEARNING OBJECTIVES

- Correlate the elements of the critical success factors for project management with the context of your DNP Project.
- Identify one key factor to carefully manage your project implementation.
- Determine the role of emotional intelligence in project management.

ACTIVITIES

Successful project management incorporates the following elements. Highlight one key area of concern in each section that may need careful management. Identify how you might address challenges that may arise for each.

Project Management Actions

- Communication
- Planning effort
- Organization
- Attention to safety and quality
- Management of project participants

Project Procedures

- Obtaining resources
- Developing an appropriate method and rollout plan

Human Factors

- Experience of participants
- Nature of the participants

- Size of organization and number of participants
- Mission/values of the organization
- Mission/values of participants

Project Factors

- Project type
- Complexity of the project
- Project timing

External Factors

- Fiscal/resource components
- Social issues
- Political issues
- System/technology issues

List three strategies to ensure success.

PROJECT PROCEDURES	HUMAN FACTORS	PROJECT FACTORS	EXTERNAL FACTORS
Identified area:	Identified area:	Identified area:	Identified area:
1.			
2.			
3.			

Tips for DNP Project Management

- Have a clear rollout plan and follow approved methodology.
- Take notes of observations and incidental comments.
- After completion of the intervention, reflect on what could be improved.
- Resolve conflicts and issues in a timely manner.
- Communicate regularly with the DNP team and project participants.
- Do not change the project method without consulting the DNP team/institutional review board (IRB).

NEXT STEPS

- Communicate regularly with your DNP team.
- Utilize the suggested tips for DNP Project management.

REFERENCES AND RESOURCES

Alias, Z., Zawawi, E. M. A., Yusof, K., & Aris, N. M. (2014). Determining critical success factors of project management practice: A conceptual framework. *Social and Behavioral Sciences, 153*, 61–69. https://doi.org/10.1016/j.sbspro.2014.10.041

Ellis, P. (2017). Learning emotional intelligence and what it can do for you. *Wounds UK, 13*(4), 66–69. https://www.wounds-uk.com

Goleman, D. (1995). *Emotional intelligence*. Bantam Books.

Mind Tools. (2019). *How emotionally intelligent are you*? https://www.mindtools.com/pages/article/ei-quiz.htm

RELATED TEXTBOOK

Broome, M. E., & Marshall, E. S. (2020). *Transformational leadership in nursing* (3rd ed.). Springer Publishing Company.

Chapter 3: Current Challenges in Complex Healthcare Organizations and the Quadruple Aim

LESSON 8.2

WRITING THE RESULTS AND DISCUSSION SECTIONS

BACKGROUND

After data collection and data analysis, you are ready to begin writing the next components of your final academic paper for the DNP Project. In most cases, you will take the DNP Project proposal, change it to past tense, and then make other revisions. Again, follow your school's specific requirements. Then you will begin to add more sections to follow the methodology section:

- Results
- Discussion
- Limitations
- Implications
- Plan for Sustainability
- Plan for Dissemination
- Conclusion

Results of the DNP Project must first be reported. Generally, the approach for reporting follows the logical or sometimes chronological order of data collection. It includes data on project outcomes and process. The key to the Results section is to be unbiased and simply report the information. Avoid the temptation to discuss the meaning of the information. That part comes later under Discussion. Tables and text are both utilized to convey the information. Read the Results section of several studies or other DNP Projects to better understand how findings are reported in text and graphically.

Discussion of the results offers the opportunity to interpret and convey meaning. In the Discussion section, start by briefly reminding the reader of the project aim(s) and objectives. Move the discussion through the order in which it is presented in the Results section. Make meaning out of the information. Does it support the findings of the literature or is it different? Were there any outliers? Now discuss limitations. Limitations are handicaps of the project. Is there a reason the sample size was small? Was there a sentinel event during the project? Try to explain why the results turned out the way they did.

LEARNING OBJECTIVES

- Organize the approach to writing the Results section.
- Organize the approach to the Discussion section and address any limitations.

ACTIVITIES

Use this outline to organize your approach to writing the DNP Project results (Sacred Heart University Library, n.d.; University of Southern California, 2019).

Structure and Approach

- Provide a short statement of context.
- Present information with a brief description.

Content

- Summarize key findings.
- Write in the past tense.
- Keep information in logical sequence.
- Use tables, charts, and figures to illustrate your findings.
- Focus on findings that are important.

Avoid common pitfalls in scholarly writing

- Be factual and concise.
- Present the information once.
- Save interpretation for the discussion section.

Outline your approach to writing your Results section.

Use this outline to organize your approach to writing your Discussion section.

Structure and Approach

- Use the past tense.
- Follow a logical approach.
- Use subheadings if appropriate to organize themes.

Content

- Reiterate the project problem.
- Explain key results and explain why they are important.
- Make connections between your findings and findings in the literature.
- Discuss limitations, lessons learned, and the evaluation of the DNP Project process.
- Make recommendations for future quality improvement, practice change, or research.

Problems to Avoid

- Do not introduce new results.
- Do not waste sentences restating your results.
- Do not omit negative information; present it in an objective way.

Outline your approach to writing your Discussion section.

NEXT STEPS

- Draft your DNP Project Results and Discussion sections.
- Review the draft with your DNP team.

REFERENCES AND RESOURCES

Quinn, C. T., & Rush, A. J. (2009, June). Writing and publishing your research findings. *Journal of Investigative Medicine, 57*(5), 634–639. https://doi.org/10.231/JIM.0b013e3181aa089f

Sacred Heart University Library. (n.d.). *Organizing academic research papers: 7. The results.* https://library.sacredheart.edu/c.php?g =29803&p=185931

University of Southern California. (2019). *Research guides. Organizing your social sciences research paper: 7. The results.* https://libguides.usc.edu/writingguide/results

LESSON 8.3

WRITING ABOUT IMPACT AND IMPLICATIONS

BACKGROUND

The complexity of the healthcare system has put patients, families, and populations at risk (Institute of Medicine, 2000). The DNP degree involves a skill set to equip you to make practice changes that improve the quality and safety of healthcare for the target population. The project should improve health outcomes. The work of this project must culminate in your description of the impact you have made on the selected outcomes. What are the implications of your work for the population?

The DNP Project should be designed to make an impact, directly or indirectly, on health outcomes of the targeted population (American Association of Colleges of Nursing [AACN], 2015). The DNP Project could also make an impact on other related components of the healthcare environment. In the final academic write-up, it is important to address the project implications beyond those of the target population. The DNP Project offers an opportunity for the DNP student to demonstrate a skill set based on the DNP Essentials (AACN, 2021).

LEARNING OBJECTIVES

- Inventory the impact your DNP Project has made for patients, families, and populations.
- Draft a paragraph(s) summarizing your points.
- Explain the impact of the DNP Project on practice, education, policy, and health systems.
- Incorporate this information into the final academic write-up.

ACTIVITIES

Reflect on the outcomes of your DNP Project.

Describe the impact it has made for patients, families, and populations.

Do you have direct quotes from your data that are significant?

Did you make observations during the intervention that were meaningful?

After your reflection, draft a paragraph summarizing your points.

_____
_____
_____
_____
_____
_____
_____
_____
_____
_____
_____

ACTIVITIES

For each category, explain the impact on your DNP Project.

Impact on Practice	Impact on Education
Impact on Policy	**Impact on Health Systems**

NEXT STEPS

- Based on your notes here, translate the information into a dedicated section of the final DNP Project write-up.

REFERENCES

American Association of Colleges of Nursing. (2015). *The doctor of nursing practice: Current issues and clarifying recommendations [White paper]*. https://www.aacnnursing.org/Portals/42/News/White-Papers/DNP-Implementation-TF-Report-8-15.pdf

American Association of Colleges of Nursing. (2021). *The essentials: Core competencies for professional nursing education*. https://www.aacnnursing.org/Portals/0/PDFs/Publications/Essentials-2021.pdf

Kohn, L. T., Corrigan, J. M., & Donaldson, M. S. (Eds.). (2000). *To err is human: Building a safer health system*. National Academies Press.

LESSON 8.4

COMPLETING THE FINAL ACADEMIC PAPER

BACKGROUND

The final academic paper of the DNP Project will vary depending on the requirements of the given program. In most cases, the document evolves from small, tangible tasks to a completed report describing the findings and implications. Because it is written in sections over time, it typically builds until one final academic paper is completed. The intended audience for this paper is the DNP faculty and other academic colleagues. It is an academic product that includes components to demonstrate DNP program outcomes.

Later, as you prepare to publish the findings of your DNP Project, the paper will need to be revised. Findings of quality-improvement projects are often written using the Standards for QUality Improvement Reporting Excellence (SQUIRE) 2.0 Guidelines (Ogrinc et al., 2016). Key information may need to be de-identified and removed. Some components of the paper that are necessary for academia are not necessary for a journal. It is important to streamline the content.

LEARNING OBJECTIVES

- Compare the SQUIRE 2.0 Guidelines to the requirements for the final academic paper at your school.
- Dissect the differences in writing for academic purposes versus for a journal audience.

ACTIVITIES

Review the requirements for the final academic paper at your school. Compare the requirements to the SQUIRE 2.0 Guidelines.

REQUIREMENTS AT YOUR SCHOOL: FINAL ACADEMIC PAPER	SQUIRE 2.0 GUIDELINES
	Title
	Abstract
	Problem description
	Available knowledge
	Rationale
	Specific aims
	Context
	Intervention
	Study of the intervention
	Measures
	Analysis
	Ethical considerations
	Results
	Summary
	Interpretation
	Limitations
	Conclusion
	Funding

NEXT STEP

- Discuss the strategy for your final academic paper with your DNP team.

REFERENCE AND RESOURCE

Ogrinc, G., Davies, L., Goodman, D., Batalden, P., Davidoff, F., & Stevens, D. (2016). SQUIRE 2.0 (Standards for Quality Improvement Reporting Excellence): Revised publication guidelines from a detailed consensus process. *BMJ Quality & Safety, 25*(12), 986–992. https://doi.org/10.1136/bmjqs-2015-004411

RELATED TEXTBOOK

White, K. M., Dudley-Brown, S., & Terhaar, M. F (Eds.). (2020). *Translation of evidence into nursing and healthcare* (3rd ed.). Springer Publishing Company.

LESSON 8.5

SKILLS FOR ORAL PRESENTATIONS

BACKGROUND

Doctor of Nursing Practice (DNP) students are required to disseminate the findings of their project in multiple ways. Oral presentations to various groups is a typical requirement. Therefore, DNP students benefit from practicing and honing public speaking skills. In preparing for oral presentations, consider the target audience and the environment (Federal Emergency Management Agency, 2014). The oral presentation delivers the same content as the written paper in a more concise way.

LEARNING OBJECTIVE

- Outline strategies for effective oral presentations.

Reflection

- In the past, what have been your strengths when giving oral presentations?
- In the past, what have been your biggest challenges or weaknesses when giving oral presentations?

ACTIVITIES

Complete the prompts to organize a strategy for an effective oral presentation based on your DNP Project.

PLANNING	NOTES
- Who is the audience? - What is the purpose of the presentation? - How much time do you have? - What is the environment like?	
Outline and Visual Materials - Create an outline of your oral presentation. - Most often, the outline follows the headings in your paper. - Do not use large paragraphs and complete sentences; keep the text focused and present using bullets. - List key points.	

Practice

- Practice your presentation.
- Prepare a transcript if you cannot stay focused.
- Time yourself.

Feedback

- Videotape yourself for self-evaluation.
- Have a colleague observe you give the presentation.

Final Strategies for the Presentation Day

- Arrive early.
- Check audio/visual equipment.
- Have backup access to your files.
- Dress professionally.
- Be prepared for potential questions.

NEXT STEP

- Discuss your plan with your DNP team.

REFERENCE AND RESOURCE

Federal Emergency Management Agency. (2014). *Lesson 4.0: Preparing for oral presentations.* https://training.fema.gov/emiweb/is/is242b/student%20manual/sm_04.pdf

RELATED TEXTBOOK

White, K. M., Dudley-Brown, S., & Terhaar, M. F (Eds.). (2020). *Translation of evidence into nursing and healthcare* (3rd ed.). Springer Publishing Company.

LESSON 8.6

STRATEGIES FOR CREATING SCHOLARLY POSTERS

BACKGROUND

A poster is a concise, visual summary of your DNP Project. Scholarly posters empower DNP students to kindle important *networking* connections and *communicate* critical translation of science into practice initiatives. To promote productive networking alliances, a poster must be visually interesting to capture a conference attendee's curiosity. Conference attendees are seldom interested in posters that serve as a storehouse for massive amounts of technical verbiage and data analyses. Wise DNP students carefully select poster information and visuals that entice attendees to stop and view their posters. Once an attendee is attracted to a DNP student's project, the poster must serve as a conversation starter. As attendees begin to view a poster, the DNP student should mention the project's most important outcome, which enables the attendee to place the DNP Project into a meaningful context. This is the point at which you succinctly state your project's take-home message. For example: *From the literature, we learned that grit and social interaction are the biggest predictors for completing DNP programs and subsequently designed an intervention that helps DNP students maximize grit and social capacity.* At this point, you have provided just enough information to encourage the attendee to talk and ask questions.

LEARNING OBJECTIVES

- Design an effective scholarly poster based on your DNP Project.

Reflection

When developing a poster, who is the intended audience? Where will the poster be displayed? Are there specific requirements from the conference/event on the size or poster design?

ACTIVITIES

Because the purpose of a poster is to encourage networking and stimulate professional conversation, it is counterproductive when posters are burdened with an abundance of words impossible to pronounce, let alone define; passive tense; and convoluted structure. These drawbacks are easily avoidable by following a few simple tips about poster sections and design.

Sections

Organize your poster into seven sections (Figure 8.1):

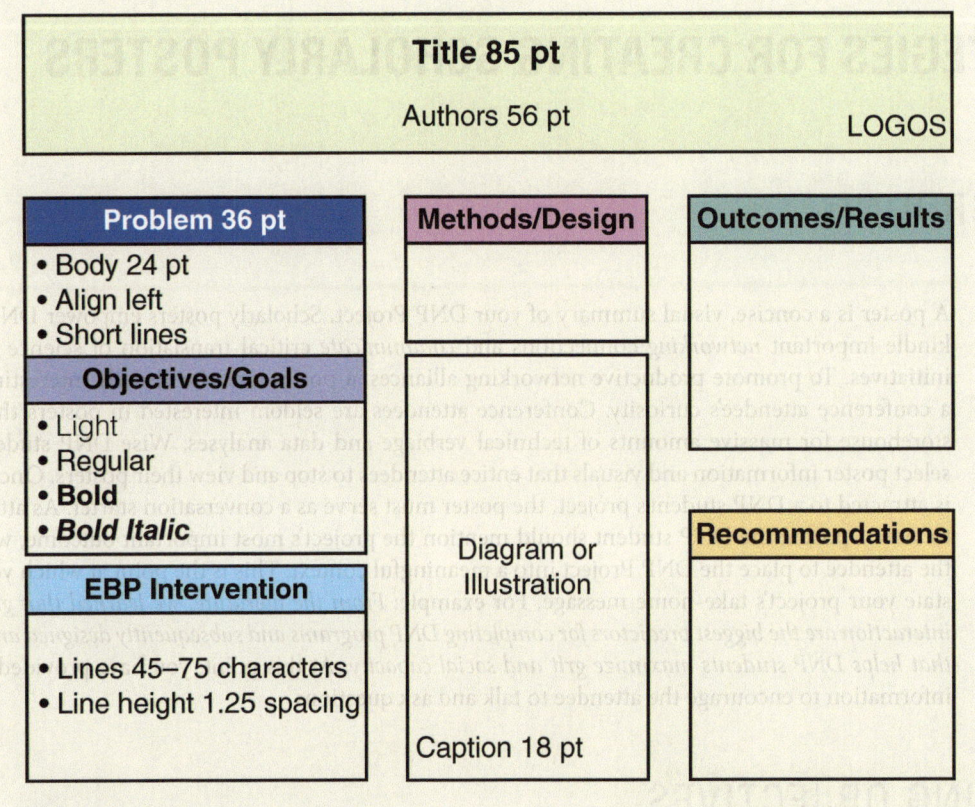

Figure 8.1 Poster design template.
Source: Reproduced from Christenbery, T. (Ed.). (2018). *Evidence-based practice in nursing* (Figure 11.3). Springer Publishing Company.

Poster template contents:
- Title 85 pt
- Authors 56 pt
- LOGOS
- **Problem 36 pt**
  - Body 24 pt
  - Align left
  - Short lines
- **Objectives/Goals**
  - Light
  - Regular
  - **Bold**
  - ***Bold Italic***
- **EBP Intervention**
  - Lines 45–75 characters
  - Line height 1.25 spacing
- **Methods/Design**
- Diagram or Illustration
- Caption 18 pt
- **Outcomes/Results**
- **Recommendations**

Section I: Title

- A title is often the first feature of the poster an attendee sees. The title needs to be large, bold, and easy to read.
- Aim for a likable title. For example: "Comfort vs. Fear: The ICU Experience" instead of "Experiences of Critically Ill Cardiac Patients: Focus Group Findings About Fear and Quality of Life."
- A title rule of thumb: *Less is more*. That is, be judicious in your selection of words for the title.
- The title header should include your name, credentials, and name of the school or organization.

Section II: Clinical Problem and Key Objectives

- Must be brief and convey the project's importance.
- Limit to two or three key objectives and relate them directly to the problem statement.
- State key objectives unambiguously and write them in bullet form.

Section III: Description of Patients, Setting, and Project

- Include important clinical and demographic data for patients.
- Briefly describe the sample selection.
- List major steps taken to implement the project and *brief* rationalizations for taking those steps.
- Describe measurement tools in this section and how data were collected.

Section IV: Outcomes and Clinical Relevance

- This is the section most attendees find of maximum interest—the so what!
- Display data analysis in this section with judicious use of charts, graphs, and pictures.
- Do not overwhelm with visuals. Generally, two graphs or charts are sufficient to display analyses.

Section V: Primary Conclusions

- State the importance of your work as a whole.
- Emphasize nursing implications and direction for future collaborative work.

Section VI: References

- Reference all sources, including images and graphs.

Section VII: Acknowledgments

- Thank those who contributed to your project. DNP work is not accomplished in a vacuum. This might include faculty advisor, institution, or funding sponsors.

Design

- **Organization:** Adhere to conference guidelines for layout (e.g., vertical, horizontal) and size. Leave space at the edges; this will help the poster to seem less cluttered. Remember, 40% of the poster should be blank or negative space. Viewers need to rest their eyes, and the negative space helps fulfill that purpose.
- **Flow:** Readers appreciate the logical flow of content. Avoid visual confusion. Use numbered headers and/or arrows to help the reader follow the intended flow. In Western countries, people generally read left to right and top to bottom. Use large, easy-to-read, and numbered sections for each of the content areas.

- **Visuals:** Use recognizable images that draw the viewer toward the poster. A recognizable image prevents your poster from looking like a wall of text. People are not interested in reading large amounts of text. If you have placed over 250 words in any section, you are way over your word count. Remember, 40% of the poster needs to be clear space.
- **Color:** Use a limited number of colors, no more than three to five, and use those colors throughout the poster, including the graphs. Use two or three primary colors and an accent color that is noticeable. The accent color should draw the viewer's eye to what you want the viewer to see.
- **Background:** No matter how amazing the photo—do not blow it up and use it for the background. Photo backgrounds are very distracting and eliminate all negative space.
- **Fonts:** Much like colors, the fewer used, the better. Only use one or two different fonts. A boldface title and headers should be 150 to 250 points, and body text uses a minimum of 48 points. The goal is to read the poster content from 3 to 4 feet. Avoid ornate lettering. A sans serif typeface, such as Arial or Helvetica, is more legible from a distance. Dark lettering on soft backgrounds is easiest to read.
- **Bullets:** Avoid making your poster look like a scholarly paper. Even a 200-word narrative placed on a poster is mind-numbing. Use bullets liberally to emphasize the salient points—they provide an easier and friendlier read for your viewer. Remember, the poster is a visual message, and it is counterproductive to insert a lengthy 200-word narrative into it.

NEXT STEP

- Design a scholarly poster based on your DNP Project.

REFERENCE AND RESOURCE

Christenbery, T. (Ed.). (2018). *Evidence-based practice in nursing.* Springer Publishing Company.

RELATED TEXTBOOK

Christenbery, T. (Ed.). (2018). *Evidence-based practice in nursing.* Springer Publishing Company.
   Chapter 11: Organizing and Evidence-Based Implementation Plan

LESSON 8.7

DNP PROJECT REPOSITORIES

BACKGROUND

The American Association of Colleges of Nursing (AACN, 2015) recommends a summary of DNP Project findings be shared beyond the academic setting. DNP students and faculty should encourage the use of digital DNP Project repositories (AACN, 2015). A repository is an electronic warehouse where intellectual property can be stored. "A digital repository for DNP final projects should be used to advance nursing practice by archiving and sharing of this work and outcomes" (AACN, 2015, p. 5).

There are different types of repositories. Determine whether a repository is available and/or required by your school. If your school does not have a repository available, some are available via professional nursing organizations. As you explore the best choice for your situation, remember to include your DNP team in the conversation. It may be necessary to de-identify agency information. You may also need to consider your plans for future publication. In most cases, use of a repository is considered a "prepublication" and does not interfere with publication in academic journals. However, read the details carefully. We recommend that an abstract of the DNP Project be uploaded to a repository at a minimum.

LEARNING OBJECTIVES

- Compare options for digital repositories.
- Determine the best fit for your situation based on your school requirements.

ACTIVITIES

Does your school have a digital repository? Yes   No

What are the requirements of your DNP program regarding a repository?

_____

_____

_____

_____

✅ Explore two additional DNP Project repositories.

Virginia Henderson Global Nursing e-Repository:

- About Us: www.nursingrepository.org/about/
- Policies and Guidelines: www.nursingrepository.org/helpfulguides/

Doctors of Nursing Practice:

- About Us: www.doctorsofnursingpractice.org/about-us/
- Doctoral Project Repository: www.doctorsofnursingpractice.org/doctoral-project-repository/

Notes

Expert Commentary: DNP Project Repositories: David G. Campbell-O'Dell, DNP, APRN, FNP-BC, FAANP

The Doctoral project repository sponsored by Doctors of Nursing Practice, Inc., is an archive of curated documents. This repository is proud to accept completed projects and displays both abstracts and full projects to all site visitors. Submission of projects does not replace or presume any publication efforts. Each listing is owned by the individual who uploads the completed academic scholarly practice project. This service allows the nursing practice scholar to share ideas and work products with the scholarly practice community and general public.

Once uploaded and posted, the owner of the documents may share the URL web page address with any individual or organization desired. Each listing helps to educate patients, employers, organizations, and other stakeholders about DNP capabilities and competencies. Your posted scholarly practice doctoral project will

- Support a collaborative engagement with practice partners and employers.
- Showcase a DNP-prepared professional's impact on improving outcomes.
- Disseminate DNP-generated content for all interested in the theme, environment, and process of impacting the complex processes of healthcare delivery.
- Build a foundation for sustainable change, future practice, and the research of practice scholarship.
- Support the growth and development of DNP students in the process of developing their projects.

☑ **Based on the findings of this lesson, my tentative plan for using a repository is to:**

_____
_____
_____
_____

NEXT STEP

- Discuss your plan with your DNP team.

REFERENCE

American Association of Colleges of Nursing. (2015). *The doctor of nursing practice: Current issues and clarifying recommendations. [White paper].* https://www.aacnnursing.org/Portals/42/News/White-Papers/DNP-Implementation-TF-Report-8-15.pdf

LESSON 8.8

SOCIAL MEDIA AND ALTERNATIVE DISSEMINATION

BACKGROUND

From an academic perspective, White et al. (2020) describe the 3P's of dissemination: (a) paper, (b) poster, and (c) presentation. The American Association of Colleges of Nursing (2015) recommends some form of DNP Project dissemination occur beyond the academic setting.

LEARNING OBJECTIVES

- Describe the target users of given social media platforms.
- Consider alternative strategies for dissemination of DNP Project findings.

ACTIVITIES

Read the Pew Research Center (2021) report and the Smith and Anderson (2018) report on social media use. Consider the descriptions of each social media platform. Highlight one social media platform for potential dissemination of DNP Project findings.

Facebook	X/Twitter	Pinterest
Snapchat	YouTube	Instagram

Other:

Selected Social Media Platform: _____

Rationale for Selection: _____

Tentative Dissemination Plan: _____

☑ **Review the following types of dissemination of DNP work and highlight three strategies you would like to use to disseminate your findings.**

PRINT	PRESENTATION
Peer-reviewed journal Review of the literature for an article, project, or practice or policy change	Scholarly presentation at professional meetings
Publications in professional publications such as newsletters and special reports	Continuing-education presentations for professionals Innovative instructional methods for students
Organizational policies and procedures Website content Budgetary analysis, review of systems processes and outcomes	Continuing education for staff, benefactors, and volunteers Bulletin boards in public locations
Health education material for the public	Presentations at support groups for specific conditions, wellness presentations for community groups
Letters to the editor, elected representatives on health issues	Testimony at public meetings

PRINT	PRESENTATION
Digital media	
Blogs, websites maintained	Videos—YouTube, Vimeo Maintain a board on Pinterest Facebook page X/Twitter feed
Social media: Facebook, X/Twitter, Instagram, Tumblr, Reddit, etc.	SlideShare Infographic
eBooks and other electronic media	Public domain photos in repositories
Broadcast	
Social media streaming Periscope Blab Facebook streaming Google Hangouts	Television interviews Radio interviews Podcast interviews Podcasts
Performances	
Poetry Fiction Drawing Photographic exhibit	Theater performances Song
Reflective and Process Oriented	

Description of process of preparing, completing DNP
Return on investment
Return on expectations
	Lessons learned regarding:
	    Working, getting an education, having a family
	    What happened after the degree?
	    Was it worth it?

Other	
Grant applications Quality reports	Travel project to apply principles in the field

Source: From Smith-Stoner, M. (2018). *A guide to disseminating your DNP project.* Springer Publishing Company.

NEXT STEP

- Discuss your plan with your DNP team.

REFERENCES AND RESOURCES

American Association of Colleges of Nursing. (2015). *The doctor of nursing practice: Current issues and clarifying recommendations. [White paper]*. https://www.aacnnursing.org/Portals/42/News/White-Papers/DNP-Implementation-TF-Report-8-15.pdf

Pew Research Center. (2021, April 7). *Social media fact sheets*. https://www.pewresearch.org/internet/fact-sheet/social-media/

Smith, A., & Anderson, M. (2018). *Social media use in 2018*. https://www.pewinternet.org/2018/03/01/social-media-use-in-2018

White, K. M., Dudley-Brown, S., & Terhaar, M. F (Eds.). (2020). *Translation of evidence into nursing and healthcare* (3rd ed.). Springer Publishing Company.

RELATED TEXTBOOK

Smith-Stoner, M. (2018). *A guide to disseminating your DNP project*. Springer Publishing Company.

Unit 1: Planning Your Dissemination Strategy
Unit 2: Introducing Types of Dissemination Methods
Unit 3: Disseminating Your Work via Print Methods
Unit 4: Disseminating Your Work via Oral Presentation Methods
Unit 5: Disseminating Work via Art and Performance Methods
Unit 6: This Is the Beginning

CHAPTER SUMMARY

Completing the work in this chapter is a major achievement! As you take these lessons and apply them to your DNP work, utilize these lessons to stay organized.

NOTES

9

The DNP Experience

Editor: Molly Bradshaw
Contributors: Tracy R. Vitale and Irina Benenson

Lessons

Lesson 9.1 Understanding the DNP Experience Hours

Lesson 9.2 American Association of Colleges of Nursing Essential Subcompetency Outliers

Lesson 9.3 Creating a DNP Portfolio

Lesson 9.4 Honing Your Political Awareness and Engagement

Lesson 9.5 Developing Business Skills

Lesson 9.6 Data Visualization

Lesson 9.7 DNP Engagement in Research and Systematic Review

Lesson 9.8 Developing Your Qualifications as a Nurse Educator

Lesson 9.9 Safety and Preparedness Skill Development

Lesson 9.10 Just Culture and the DNP Project

Lesson 9.11 Inclusion of Interprofessional Interactions

OBJECTIVES

The purpose of this chapter is to suggest potential activities for the DNP experience and beyond. The lessons related to the activities may be relevant at different points of the DNP Project process depending on the nature of the project and trajectory of the DNP curriculum. They may also contain ideas that extend beyond graduation. Consult with your faculty for further clarification on the DNP practice experience at your school. By the end of this chapter, you will be able to

- Understand the requirements for the DNP experience at your school.
- Incorporate the lessons and suggested activities into the DNP experience.
- Refer to these resources post-DNP graduation.

INTRODUCTION

According to the American Association of Colleges of Nursing (AACN, 2006, 2015, 2021), the nurse completing the DNP degree must complete a minimum of 1,000 practice hours beyond the BSN degree in order to achieve the desired outcomes. These DNP experience hours must be part of a supervised academic program. Students will often get credit for hours earned during a master's degree in nursing program. For students completing BSN–DNP programs, the hours are often collective, spent on both learning your new nursing role and completion of DNP-related work. We recommend clarifying your school's requirements.

The hours spent toward application of the *Essentials* and/or the DNP Project should be referred to as the "DNP practice experience" or "practice hours" (AACN, 2015). The faculty are responsible for assessing the needs of the students and determining the nature of the experience. The AACN (2021) notes that the immersion experience should allow for application and integration of the essential sub-competencies. The DNP practice experience should provide unique perspectives of the healthcare system, be nontraditional, be interprofessional, and expand the skill set of the DNP student. Work hours do not count, and students should not receive "credit" for years of experience (AACN, 2015). The goal is to expand horizons. Both faculty and students should carefully read the content of the AACN (2015) white paper regarding the practice experience, practice hours, and collaborative partnerships.

Because the DNP experience is widely interpreted, it begs the question, "What can I do to complete the required DNP experience hours?" The work of completing the DNP Project accounts for a good majority of the hours. However, the purpose of this chapter is to offer a series of lessons that guide you through potential activities that may contribute to your DNP experience. It is important to track all of the time spent on activities that are related to both your DNP Project and the *Essentials*. We are often asked if reading, writing, or spending time at the library counts. It may be reasonable to include a small, predetermined number of hours toward these activities. *This is up to your faculty and the policies at your school.*

We kick off this chapter by making a bold statement. Remember, you are completing a *doctoral* degree in nursing. Devoting numerous hours to reading, writing, and investigating literature is a natural expectation. *Move* beyond *these activities.* Get out and engage in some aspect of healthcare, learning, or the community that you have not explored. Several suggestions are offered. Short descriptions in the words of DNP students regarding their DNP practice experiences are found in the Chapter Summary. A log to help you track your DNP experience hours is found in the Appendix. Let's begin.

REFERENCES AND RESOURCES

American Association of Colleges of Nursing. (2006). *The essentials of doctoral education for advanced nursing practice.* https://www.aacnnursing.org/Portals/42/Publications/DNPEssentials.pdf

American Association of Colleges of Nursing. (2015). *The doctor of nursing practice: Current issues and clarifying recommendations. [White paper].* https://www.aacnnursing.org/Portals/42/News/White-Papers/DNP-Implementation-TF-Report-8-15.pdf

American Association of Colleges of Nursing. (2021). *The essentials: Core competencies for professional nursing education.* https://www.aacnnursing.org/Portals/0/PDFs/Publications/Essentials-2021.pdf

MY GOALS FOR THE DNP EXPERIENCE ARE TO:

LESSON 9.1

UNDERSTANDING THE DNP EXPERIENCE HOURS

BACKGROUND

As part of your program, you will complete a minimum of 1,000 clinical or "DNP experience" hours. These include clinical hours and the time put toward your DNP Project. As you consider your DNP practice experience, it is important to recognize what your school will allow. Some are very prescriptive, whereas others allow you to individualize your hours and have more leeway as long as your project aligns with the American Association of Colleges of Nursing (AACN) *Essentials*.

DNP experience hours may be led by either a preceptor, a faculty member, or both. For example, your DNP faculty may assign you the task of completing an interprofessional interview relevant to your DNP Project. The time would be counted toward your experience hours. Or you may be asked to complete activities in collaboration with a preceptor in a clinical site. Clarify with your faculty the expectations at your school.

The AACN (2015) suggests that DNP experiences extend beyond direct patient care. This may include indirect care practices, including larger organizations (i.e., Red Cross, organizational information technology departments, community health organizations, long-term care facilities, urgent care facilities, prisons, school systems, public health, nongovernment agencies, or private corporations). In addition to having a precepted experience, it is possible that one of these locations may also be able to translate to the site for the DNP Project (AACN, 2015).

When considering practice experiences, learning objectives should align with the DNP *Essentials* and application of theory and evidence to practice (AACN, 2015). DNP practice experiences are a great opportunity for the student to interact and collaborate interprofessionally in order to facilitate leadership and communication. The AACN (2015) outlines that the DNP program practice experiences should provide:

- Systematic opportunities for feedback and reflection.
- In-depth work/mentorship with experts in nursing, as well as other disciplines.
- Opportunities for meaningful student engagement within practice environments.
- Opportunities for building and assimilating knowledge for advanced nursing practice at a high level of complexity.
- Opportunities for further application, synthesis, and expansion of learning.
- Experience in the context of advanced nursing practice within which the final DNP Project is completed.
- Opportunities for integrating and synthesizing all of the DNP *Essentials* and role requirements necessary to demonstrate achievement of defined outcomes in an area of advanced nursing practice.

LEARNING OBJECTIVES

- Describe acceptable DNP hours based on the policies of your DNP Project.
- Distinguish between preceptor-led and faculty-led DNP hours.

ACTIVITIES

Outline the requirements related to DNP experience hours at your school. List key points here.

_____
_____
_____

Are there any limitations on the requirements of a precepted DNP experience set forth by your academic institution?

_____
_____
_____

What are your skill development needs:

_____
_____
_____

What will you need to help you develop, implement, and evaluate your DNP Project?

_____
_____
_____

Who in your professional network may be able to work with you during your DNP experience?

_____
_____
_____

NEXT STEPS

- List any questions you have for your DNP chair.
- Confirm the DNP experience activity with faculty early in the process.

REFERENCES AND RESOURCES

American Association of Colleges of Nursing. (2006). *The essentials of doctoral education for advanced nursing practice*. https://wwwaacnnursing.org/Portals/42/Publications/DNPEssentials.pdf

American Association of Colleges of Nursing. (2015). *The doctor of nursing practice: Current issues and clarifying recommendations*. [White paper]. https://www.aacnnursing.org/Portals/42/News/White-Papers/DNP-Implementation-TF-Report-8-15.pdf

American Association of Colleges of Nursing. (2021). *The essentials: Core competencies for professional nursing education*. https://www.aacnnursing.org/Portals/0/PDFs/Publications/Essentials-2021.pdf

LESSON 9.2

AMERICAN ASSOCIATION OF COLLEGES OF NURSING ESSENTIAL SUBCOMPETENCY OUTLIERS

BACKGROUND

All *Essentials* should be met by the end of the DNP program. The DNP Project provides the student with an opportunity to operationalize skills and demonstrate competency. Each domain of the *Essentials* (2021) has a list of sub-competencies. Take this opportunity to identify outliers. What has been met through the work of your project? What is still outstanding?

LEARNING OBJECTIVE

- Identify opportunities to meet American Association of Colleges of Nursing (AACN) sub-competencies.

ACTIVITIES

In Chapter 2, you examined the DNP Project as it relates to the AACN *Essentials* and sub-competencies. Now, use the same list to review and identify any potential gaps. Are there any competencies you have not met or will not meet? If yes, plan a dedicated activity.

Domain 1: Knowledge for Nursing Practice

Sub-competencies Met:

Gaps:

Planned Activity to Fill Gap:

Domain 2: Person-Centered Care

Sub-competencies Met:

Gaps:

Planned Activity to Fill Gap:

Domain 3: Population Health

Sub-competencies Met:

Gaps:

Planned Activity to Fill Gap:

Domain 4: Scholarship for Nursing Practice

Sub-competencies Met:

Gaps:

Planned Activity to Fill Gap:

Domain 5: Quality and Safety

Sub-competencies Met:

Gaps:

Planned Activity to Fill Gap:

Domain 6: Interprofessional Partnerships

Sub-competencies Met:

Gaps:

Planned Activity to Fill Gap:

Domain 7: Systems-Based Practice

Sub-competencies Met:

Gaps:

Planned Activity to Fill Gap:

Domain 8: Informatics and Healthcare Technologies

Sub-competencies Met:

Gaps:

Planned Activity to Fill Gap:

Domain 9: Professionalism

Sub-competencies Met:

Gaps:

Planned Activity to Fill Gap:

Domain 10: Personal, Professional, and Leadership Development

Sub-competencies Met:

Gaps:

Planned Activity to Fill Gap:

NEXT STEP

Questions from faculty/DNP chair regarding DNP project experience log:
_____
_____
_____

REFERENCES AND RESOURCES

American Association of Colleges of Nursing. (2006). *The essentials of doctoral education for advanced nursing practice.* https://www.aacnnursing.org/Portals/42/Publications/DNPEssentials.pdf

American Association of Colleges of Nursing. (2021). *The essentials: Core competencies for professional nursing education.* https://www.aacnnursing.org/Education-Resources/AACN-Essentials

LESSON 9.3

CREATING A DNP PORTFOLIO

BACKGROUND

A DNP portfolio is a collection of your work that showcases different assignments or elements of your doctoral scholarship. It could be used to demonstrate learning outcomes (DNP *Essentials*) presented during a job interview or included as a part of your current promotion/tenure procedure. The DNP portfolio is not a substitution for a DNP Project (American Association of Colleges of Nursing [AACN], 2015).

Before you develop a DNP portfolio, consider its purpose and intended audience. Determine whether the DNP portfolio will be organized in hard copy or electronically. If it is electronic, consider whether you will be able to access it beyond graduation. Remember that certain information or assignments may need to be de-identified if it is accessible by the public.

LEARNING OBJECTIVES

- Determine the purpose and intended audience.
- Identify the components of the portfolio.
- Ensure safe-keeping of sensitive information.
- Explore the options for creating a dedicated website.

ACTIVITIES

Complete these prompts.

DNP portfolio:

- Purpose:
- Intended audience:
- List potential items to include:
  - Assignments?
  - Unique or creative work?
  - DNP Project executive summary?
  - Other
  - Consider mapping content to the DNP *Essentials*

☑ **Maintaining a website-based DNP portfolio is an excellent way to ensure that your portfolio is easily accessible. There are several companies that offer free capabilities for creating websites. One of our favorites is WIX.com. Explore their services (www.wix.com).**

Review these examples of DNP portfolios:

- https://npmollyb.wixsite.com/who4nprx
- https://tracyvitalednp.wixsite.com/mysite
- https://aleksandranovik.wixsite.com/cdsmonitoringtools/dnp-project
- https://depaul.digication.com/linda_a_graf_dnp_portfolio/Welcome/published

NEXT STEPS

- Discuss your plan with your DNP team and DNP faculty.
- Develop a DNP portfolio.

REFERENCES AND RESOURCES

American Association of Colleges of Nursing. (2015). *The doctor of nursing practice: Current issues and clarifying recommendations. [White paper].* https://www.aacnnursing.org/Portals/42/News/White-Papers/DNP-Implementation-TF-Report-8-15.pdf

American Association of Colleges of Nursing. (2021). *The essentials: Core competencies for professional nursing education.* https://www.aacnnursing.org/Education-Resources/AACN-Essentials

Havercamp, J., & Vogt, M. (2015). Beyond academic evidence: Uses of technology within e-portfolio for the doctor of nursing practice program. *Journal of Professional Nursing, 31*(4), 284–289. https://doi.org/10.1016/j.profnurs.2015.03.007

Melander, S., Hardin-Pierce, M., & Ossage, J. (2018). Development of a rubric for evaluation of the DNP portfolio. *Nursing Education Perspectives, 39*(5), 312–314. https://doi.org/10.1097/01.NEP.0000000000000381

University of Arizona. (2019). *DNP portfolio.* https://www.nursing.arizona.edu/resources/dnp-portfolio

RELATED TEXTBOOK

Smith-Stoner, M. (2018). *A guide to disseminating your DNP project.* Springer Publishing Company.

LESSON 9.4

HONING YOUR POLITICAL AWARENESS AND ENGAGEMENT

BACKGROUND

Awareness and engagement in policy development are key to changing health outcomes. DNP-prepared nurses should have skill sets to become influential in policy conversation, otherwise nursing influence on policy is lost. Without influence, our ability to transform care is limited (Dreher & Smith Glasgow, 2017). Many nursing organizations also have policy/advocacy information available on their website. The American Nurses Association (n.d.) has an Advocacy Toolkit Policy; National League for Nursing (n.d.) has an Advocacy Action Center where you can sign up for alerts, identify/contact legislators, and follow current legislation.

EXPERT COMMENTARY: UNDERSTANDING THE ROLE OF THE DNP IN HEALTH POLICY

During our doctoral education, we were challenged as students to identify key policy makers. What was originally perceived to be a civic lesson quickly turned into a reality check. When the class was presented with the headshots of some obviously recognizable figures like the president of the United States and the state governor, overall confidence quickly decreased as images of our state senators, local representatives, and other key players, including the U.S. Secretary of Health and Human Services and chair of the Institute of Medicine committee on the Future of Nursing, were presented and we did not know who they were.

As nurses, especially those with a DNP, it is our obligation not only to be aware but also to be active in health policy. This may include working within an organization at the local, state, or national level. Regardless of our intended roles, our lawmakers are guiding the way we practice. On a state level, legislators are currently making decisions on topics, including a joint protocol with physicians, a multistate nurse licensure compact, nurse staffing ratios, requiring newly licensed RNs to attain a BSN within 10 years of initial licensure as a condition of license renewal, minimal staffing, and other legislation impacting nurses and overall healthcare delivered.

—Tracy R. Vitale

LEARNING OBJECTIVES

- Identify key policy makers in your geographic area.
- Identify current state legislation impacting nurses/the nursing profession.
- Develop a letter to a local/state representative on a healthcare topic of interest.

ACTIVITIES

1. Using the website links, identify your representative and their contact information:
    State governor: www.usa.gov/state-governor

    U.S. senators: www.senate.gov/general/contact_information/senators_cfm.cfm

    U.S. representative: www.house.gov/representatives/find-your-representative

    Federal, state, and local representatives: www.usa.gov/elected-officials

2. Identify the names of the people in the following positions in your state/area:
    State governor

    U.S. senator:

    U.S. senator:

    National representative:

    National representative:

    Local representative (state senator/assembly/etc.):

    Local representative (state senator/assembly/etc.):

3. Using the information collected, navigate your state's legislative website and identify a bill currently being considered. Review the bill, identify any groups that are supporting/opposing the bill, and determine your stance. Once you have done this, draft a letter to the appropriate representative supporting/opposing the bill using the following sites as samples for templates:
    https://www.ncsbn.org/APRN_formletter_Legislator_web.pdf

    http://www.nea.org/home/19657.htm

    http://advocacy.aone.org/legislative-basics/how-communicate-and-build-relationship-your-legislators

NEXT STEPS

- Identify political/advocacy efforts being done by any of your professional organizations.
- Discuss with your mentors/leaders any advocacy they have been involved in.

REFERENCES AND RESOURCES

American Association of Nurse Practitioners. (n.d.). *Championing the NP role and amplifying the NP voice.* https://www.aanp.org/advocacy

American Nurses Association. (n.d.). *ANA advocacy toolkit.* https://www.nursingworld.org/practice-policy/advocacy/ana-advocacy-toolbox/

American Organization for Nursing Leadership. (2019). *How to communicate with your legislators.* http://advocacy.aone.org/legislative-basics/how-communicate-and-build-relationship-your-legislators

Dreher, H. M., & Smith Glasgow, M. E. (2017). *DNP role development for doctoral advanced nursing practice* (2nd ed.). Springer Publishing Company.

HHS.gov. (n.d.). *About the affordable care act.* https://www.hhs.gov/healthcare/about-the-aca/index.html

National Council of State Boards of Nursing. (n.d.). *Template letter to a legislator.* https://www.ncsbn.org/APRN_formletter_Legislator_web.pdf

National Education Association. (n.d.). *Writing to your legislators.* http://www.nea.org/home/19657.htm

National League for Nursing. (n.d.). *Advocacy action center.* http://www.nln.org/advocacy-public-policy/legislative-issues

RELATED TEXTBOOK

Dreher, H. M., & Smith Glasgow, M. E. (2017). *DNP role development for doctoral advanced nursing practice* (2nd ed.). Springer Publishing Company.

LESSON 9.5

DEVELOPING BUSINESS SKILLS

BACKGROUND

The DNP Project is an opportunity for students to develop business competencies. For example, do you have an ability to engage in fiscal conversations? Managing department budgets and participating in conversations related to reimbursements are natural expectations. In fact, as a DNP experience, spending time with the organization's chief financial officer may provide some unique insight. In another example, consider the idea of marketing. "Marketing" is a term used to describe a series of activities designed to create buy-in among consumers. The consumer may be seeking information, services, or a product. However, there is definite skill and science involved in the process. Effective marketing helps others understand the abilities of DNP-prepared nurses and engages our patients, staff, stakeholders, and other "consumers" in our products and services. Creating a clear marketing message is the first step. These are just two examples of business skills.

Review the recommendations from the American Organization for Nurse Leaders (AONL) regarding competencies. They recommend five domains of competencies for nurse leaders: (a) Communication, (b) Knowledge, (c) Leadership, (d) Professionalism, and (e) Business Skills. Specifically mentioned in the section on business skills is a list of potential ideas including financial management, human resource management, strategic management, marketing, and information/technology (2015). We will review that document in this lesson for relevance to your project.

Beyond engagement in pre-established business, some DNP students may consider an entrepreneurial approach to the work of the DNP Project. Is there a product that you want to sell to improve health outcomes? Is there a service you want to provide? There are time limits to DNP Projects. However, developing a business plan to later launch a business could be a beneficial learning experience.

LEARNING OBJECTIVES

- Examine the AONL Leadership Competencies related to "Business Skills."
- Explore resources for writing business and marketing plans.

ACTIVITIES: AMERICAN ORGANIZATION FOR NURSE LEADERS LEADERSHIP COMPETENCIES

Visit this website and review the AONL Leadership Competencies for Population Health. Look specifically at the competencies listed under "Business Skills." Make a list of three to five items you could include as learning activities in your DNP experience.

Link: https://www.aonl.org/system/files/media/file/2019/10/population-health-competencies.pdf

1.

2.

3.

4.

5.

ACTIVITIES: BUSINESS PLANS

Business plans start with a product or service that you want to sell to a consumer. Could this relate to your DNP Project? Answer these questions:

Why do you want to start this business?

Logistics:

    Product/service offered:

    Schedule:

    Budget:

What will you charge?

What will your policies be?

Make it official:

Will there be incorporation, licensing, and so on?

How will income and expenses be tracked?

Will you need start-up funding?

Ensure proper tax withholding.

Put yourself out there:

How will you advertise your services/product?

Examples of DNP student projects turned to businesses:

- Development of a mobile app
- Development of a mobile health clinic
- Development of an online business

ACTIVITIES: MARKETING PLANS

As you work with organizations to improve health outcomes, consider the impact of marketing. Does the organization market its services well? Do you market yourself well as a professional? Use the DNP practice experience to improve your business-related marketing skills.

Donald Miller (2017) is the author of the best-selling book, *Building a StoryBrand: Clarify Your Message So Customers Will Listen*. He has developed a marketing framework that he calls the "SB7 Framework." He bases this marketing strategy on the ancient art of storytelling. He believes that by telling a story well, you create effective marketing. According to Miller, a good story starts with a character (consumer) who encounters a problem. The consumer then meets a guide (DNP student) who understands his or her fear and gives the consumer a skill, solution, or product to solve their problem. Effective marketing should always present a call to action with a clear indication of the success or failure that could occur. In the end, the consumer is the hero of the story (consumer/patient).

Go to https://storybrand.com to read more about Story Brand. Based on your DNP Project or DNP practice experience, identify an element that would benefit from effective marketing. List it here:

_____

_____

_____

If you are having difficulty thinking of a practice application, consider how you will market your DNP career when you graduate.

On the website https://storybrand.com, scroll down and complete the free 5-Minute Marketing Makeover. Based on what you learned, list three things you will do to improve the marketing of your DNP Project or practice.

1.

2.

3.

NEXT STEPS

- Discuss your plans with your DNP team.

REFERENCES AND RESOURCES

AONE, AONL. (2015). *AONL nurse manager competencies.* AONE, AONL http://www.aonl.org/

Coleman, K. (2023). *How to start a business.* Ramsey Solutions. https://www.ramseysolutions.com/business/the-basics-of-starting-a-business

Miller, D. (2017). *Building a story brand: Clarify your message so customers will listen.* Harper Collins Leadership. https://www.amazon.com/Building-StoryBrand-Clarify-Message-Customers/dp/0718033329

LESSON 9.6

DATA VISUALIZATION

BACKGROUND

The DNP Project will generate data. Consider the best approach for dissemination of the data. Will other scholars review it, or will community stakeholders and patients review it? Translating data into visual form makes it easier to understand. It is estimated that 65% of people are visual learners; the brain can process visual images 60,000 times faster than information written in words (Bradshaw & Porter, 2017). As part of the DNP practice experience, consider incorporating data visualization into your DNP Project dissemination plan.

Creating infographics and listicles are activities within the realm of data visualization. An infographic is composed of synthesized data that are visually translated, arranged in a way that tells a story, have a call to action, and are a verifiable source of information (Bradshaw & Porter, 2017). Infographics are often best suited for quantitative data. For qualitative information consider writing a listicle. A listicle is information written in a way that combines the concepts of "article" and "lists." Listicles often have a cardinal number in the title, have an opening comment, and are supported by key information in list format. At the end, there should also be a closing remark, call to action, and verifiable source of information. As a DNP student, this is a skill you should consider developing. These formats are well received online and on social media.

LEARNING OBJECTIVES

- Gather data that need to be presented.
- Investigate resources for developing an infographic or listicle.

ACTIVITIES

Infographics

A well-developed infographic should have the following:

- A standout title.
- A short, one- to two-sentence opening remark that conveys the purpose of the infographic.
- Key pieces of data and information.
- A call to action.
- A follow-up and/or place to seek additional information.

Examine this infographic. Can you identify these elements? Circle them when you find them.

Link: NPGraphicOption1_Edit15_111122 (aanp.org)

Now plan your infographic:

Title:

Opening Remark:

Data Points:

Call to Action:

Follow-Up Link:

After planning and sketching your infographics, explore these websites for creating infographics. Select the free option for infographics and use their predesigned templates to create your infographic.

- Canva: https://www.canva.com/
- Piktochart: https://piktochart.com/

Listicles

Explore these links to help you create listicles.

- Mulholland, B. (2018). *Writing a listicle: The 11 step guide and why they are awesome*. https://www.process.st/listicle/
- Shook, M. (2018). *5 simple tips for writing awesome listicles for medium*. https://medium.com/publishous/5-simple-tips-for-writing-awesome-listicles-for-medium-d3e6e7112fa6

Now plan your listicle. Write your notes. Use the same websites mentioned earlier to create yours.

Introduction

Data Point

Data Point

Data Point

Conclusion

*** HINT: Keep data points as an odd number 3, 5, 7, etc.

NEXT STEPS

- Discuss your plans with your DNP team.
- Continue to develop data visualization skills.

REFERENCES AND RESOURCES

Bradshaw, M., & Porter, S. (2017). Infographics: A new tool for the nursing classroom. *Nurse Educator, 42*(2), 57–59. https://doi.org/10.1097/nne.0000000000000316

Mulholland, B. (2018). *Writing a listicle: The 11 step guide and why they are awesome.* https://www.process.st/listicle/

Shook, M. (2018). *5 simple tips for writing awesome listicles for medium.* https://medium.com/publishous/5-simple-tips-for-writing-awesome-listicles-for-medium-d3e6e7112fa6

LESSON 9.7

DNP ENGAGEMENT IN RESEARCH AND SYSTEMATIC REVIEWS

BACKGROUND

The differences between DNP and PhD prepared nurses was explored in an earlier chapter. Although the education and roles may have very different focuses, there is a wealth of opportunity for collaboration in which each can utilize the others' strengths. One such opportunity is the ability for DNPs to engage in research and systematic reviews. The collaboration can allow for the dissemination of knowledge, scientific inquiry, and translational research (American Association of Colleges of Nursing [AACN], 2004, 2006, 2016, 2021).

Engagement in Research

In 2018, the AACN recommended that PhDs and DNPs need to partner with each other in order to translate newly generated knowledge into practices. A PhD nurse scientist, in collaboration with the DNP nurse leader, can design a study to collect data to explore variations in the clinical problem. The DNP can explore current literature for potential implementation strategies while bringing organizational leadership expertise about potential financial implications and leadership to further improve the design of the research to answer this clinical question (Trautman et al., 2018). As the PhD-prepared nurse can design an interventional study, the DNP-prepared nurse can lead the shift of changing practice based on the results of the study. DNP students could benefit from further development of research skills as a portion of their DNP experience hours.

Engagement in Systematic Review

A systematic review is often considered the basis for evidence-based practice (Holly et al., 2017). Systematic reviews can be helpful in interpreting knowledge from a large collection of studies about a particular topic or situation (Staffileno & Foreman, 2018). In a systematic review, there is a focused question and specific protocol used to identify, critique, and eventually provide a collective summary of primary research (Baker & Weeks, 2014). There are several organizations that collect and publish systematic reviews, including Campbell Collaboration, Cochrane Collaboration, and Joanna Briggs Institute. These organizations provide guidance and training, as well as the necessary computer software to support evidence synthesis (Staffileno & Foreman, 2018).

The AACN (2015) states that systematic review as a DNP Project does not allow for integrating scholarship into practice. However, a systematic review can set the stage for evidence transfer/translation and provide a DNP with a skill set to change practice. Therefore, the DNP student may benefit from engagement in systematic review as a portion of their DNP experience hours.

LEARNING OBJECTIVES

- Explore opportunities to engage in research guided by a PhD-prepared leader.
- Explore opportunities to receive training and engage in formal systematic review.

EXPERT COMMENTARY: USE OF SYSTEMATIC REVIEW IN NURSE PRACTITIONER PRACTICE

A long time ago, I read a study about what makes a good clinician. Some factors you might think were important, like grades achieved during your training, were irrelevant. What correlated the best was the number of medical journals a clinician read. I don't know whether that means good clinicians read more journals or reading more journals makes a better clinician. One thing I know is that reading and understanding medical literature requires critical analysis skills. However, it was not until I performed my first systematic review that I started to develop these skills.

Before knowing how to appraise literature, I really wasn't aware of all the things that can go wrong in a study, and I didn't know what to look for to decide whether the results were really credible. I thought the authors knew a lot more than I did, and I trusted them to a degree that was not warranted. The more I immersed myself in reviewing the literature and learned about fundamental bias of research (flaws in the process of participant selection, data collection, and interpretation), the less I was willing to be a passive absorber of information. I learned to question the results and reach my own conclusions on what the best evidence is. Literature reading skills helped me to be a better consumer of medical journals and a better clinician. Understanding studies and making clinical decisions based on valid evidence became crucial to my everyday practice of diagnosing and treating patients—which of course is the ultimate purpose of medical research.

—Irina Benenson

ACTIVITIES: ENGAGEMENT IN RESEARCH

Identify nurse researchers at your partnering agency who have a focus in your area of interest and review their publications on their work. Are there professional organizations in need of students to help with research agendas?

- Is there a component of their work you could participate in?
- How could you further partner?

ACTIVITIES: ENGAGEMENT OF SYSTEMATIC REVIEW

We have already discussed that DNPs are responsible for transferring knowledge into practice. With that said, if you find yourself able to participate in conducting a systematic review, you can bring the knowledge transfer component into play. Examples of knowledge transfer/translation options include using the results of the systematic review to

- Develop an evidence-based teaching tool.
- Develop a pilot study to implement recommendations.
- Develop or update an existing practice policy.
- Develop clinical audit criteria.

Identify a systematic review relevant to your DNP Project. Use a critical appraisal tool to review the findings. List three ways the information can be applied in practice:

1.
2.
3.

NEXT STEPS

- List any questions you have for your DNP team.
- Consider establishing a plan for future research.
- Consider additional training on the process of systematic review.

REFERENCES AND RESOURCES

American Association of Colleges of Nursing. (2004). *AACN position statement on the practice Doctorate in nursing.* Author.

American Association of Colleges of Nursing. (2006). *The essentials of doctoral education for advanced nursing practice.* Author.

American Association of Colleges of Nursing. (2016). *Advancing healthcare transformation: A new era for academic nursing.* http://www.aacnnursing.org/Portals/42/Publications/AACN-New-Era-Report.pdf

American Association of Colleges of Nursing. (2018). *Defining scholarship for academic nursing.* http://www.aacnnursing.org/News-Information/Position-Statements-White-Papers/Defining-Scholarship-Nursing

American Association of Colleges of Nursing. (2021). *The essentials: Core competencies for professional nursing education.* https://www.aacnnursing.org/Education-Resources/AACN-Essentials

Baker, K. A., & Weeks, S. M. (2014). An overview of systematic review. *Journal of PeriAnesthesia Nursing, 29*(6), 454–458. https://doi.org/10.1016/j.jopan.2014.07.002

Holly, C., Salmond, S., & Saimbert, M. (Eds.). (2017). *Comprehensive systematic review for advanced practice nursing* (2nd ed.). Springer Publishing Company.

Staffileno, B. A., & Foreman, M. D. (2018). *Research for advanced practice nurses: From evidence to practice* (3rd ed.). Springer Publishing Company.

Trautman, D. E., Idzik, S., Hammersla, M., & Rosseter, R. (2018). Advancing scholarship through translational research: The role of PhD and DNP prepared nurses. *The Online Journal of Issues in Nursing, 23*(2). https://doi.org/10.3912/OJIN.Vol23No02Man02

RELATED TEXTBOOKS

Holly, C., Salmond, S., & Saimbert, M. (Eds.). (2017). *Comprehensive systematic review for advanced practice nursing* (2nd ed.). Springer Publishing Company.

Melnyk, B. M., & Morrison-Beedy, D. (2018). *Intervention research and evidence-based quality improvement: Designing, conducting, analyzing, and funding* (2nd ed.). Springer Publishing Company.

Staffileno, B. A., & Foreman, M. D. (2018). *Research for advanced practice nurses: From evidence to practice* (3rd ed.). Springer Publishing Company.

LESSON 9.8

DEVELOPING YOUR QUALIFICATIONS AS A NURSE EDUCATOR

BACKGROUND

The DNP degree is a practice-focused doctorate (American Association of Colleges of Nursing [AACN], 2015). "Practice" is defined by the AACN (2004) as "any form of nursing intervention that influences healthcare outcomes for individuals or populations, including the direct care of individual patients, management of care for individuals and populations, administration of nursing and healthcare organizations, and the development and implementation of health policy" (p. 2).

Many students enroll in DNP programs with the intention of becoming a nurse educator in the future. The DNP degree is designed to prepare you for the highest levels of nursing practice. To be an effective nurse educator, you must first be an expert in nursing practice. Obtaining a DNP degree does make you qualified to teach. However, it does not prepare you for the faculty role. Additional training will be needed. The AACN (2015) reaffirmed previous recommendations that nursing education requires a distinct body of knowledge and competencies that are not of the same scope as the DNP degree.

If you are interested in becoming a nurse educator, you can complete additional training and coursework within the DNP program (AACN, 2015). Training in nursing education is optional and may or may not be available as part of your school or DNP curriculum. You must discuss this endeavor with your DNP faculty and DNP program director. If it is an option, this additional study may help you further add to your qualification as a nurse educator. The purpose of this lesson is to explore options for professional development in the nurse educator role offered by the National League for Nursing (NLN).

LEARNING OBJECTIVES

- Review the mission statement of the NLN.
- Examine opportunities for further development in the role of nurse educator.

ACTIVITIES

1. Visit the website of the NLN (www.nln.org). Review the NLN Vision for Doctoral Preparation of Nurse Educators (www.nln.org/docs/default-source/about/nln-vision-series-%28position-statements%29/nlnvision_6.pdf?sfvrsn=4).

NOTES

_____
_____
_____

2. Review the available professional development programs and teaching resources (www.nln.org/professional-development-programs).

NOTES

_____
_____
_____

3. Review the qualifications for certification in nursing education (CNE; www.nln.org/Certification-for-Nurse-Educators).

NOTES

☑ **Identify nurse educator opportunities at your school.**

☑ **Write a plan to develop your qualifications as a nurse educator.**

NEXT STEPS

- Discuss your plans with your DNP team.
- Continue to develop your qualifications as a nurse educator beyond graduation.

REFERENCES AND RESOURCES

American Association of Colleges of Nursing. (2004). *AACN position statement on the practice doctorate in nursing.* [White paper]. https://www.aacnnursing.org/Portals/42/News/Position-Statements/DNP.pdf

American Association of Colleges of Nursing. (2015). *The doctor of nursing practice: Current issues and clarifying recommendations.* [White paper]. https://www.aacnnursing.org/Portals/42/News/White-Papers/DNP-Implementation-TF-Report-8-15.pdf

RELATED TEXTBOOK

Dreher, H. M., & Glasgow, M. (2018). *DNP role development for doctoral advanced practice nursing.* Springer Publishing Company.

Chapter 7: The Role of the Nurse Educator

LESSON 9.9

SAFETY AND PREPAREDNESS SKILL DEVELOPMENT

BACKGROUND

Implementing projects on a large scale may involve planning for safety of the patient and the healthcare team. Safety considerations may range from use of personal protective equipment to planning for weather. The American Association of Colleges of Nursing (AACN) 2021 Essentials and Healthy People 2030 specifically mention emergency preparedness as important to social determinants of health and the skill set of DNP leaders.

The Federal Emergency Management Association (FEMA) has numerous resources for use in healthcare. They also discuss the National Preparedness Goal as addressing five key mission areas:

- **Prevention:** Prevent, avoid, or stop an imminent, threatened, or actual act of terrorism.
- **Protection**: Protect our citizens, residents, visitors, and assets against the greatest threats and hazards in a manner that allows our interests, aspirations, and way of life to thrive.
- **Mitigation**: Reduce the loss of life and property by lessening the impact of future disasters.
- **Response**: Respond quickly to save lives; protect property and the environment; and meet basic human needs in the aftermath of an incident.
- **Recovery**: Recover through a focus on the timely restoration, strengthening, and revitalization of infrastructure, housing, and a sustainable economy, as well as the health, social, cultural, historic, and environmental fabric of communities affected by an incident. The mission areas and core capabilities organize the community-wide activities and tasks performed before, during, and after disasters into a framework for achieving the goal of a secure and resilient Nation (FEMA, 2018).

In developing your skill set as a nurse leader, consider spending some of your DNP experience hours engaging in community assessments or organizational assessments relevant to emergency preparedness. How could an emergency impact your DNP Project?

LEARNING OBJECTIVES

- Review FEMA recommendations related to your organization and population.
- Determine organizational needs during emergency response.
- Plan for emergencies/contingencies that may arise during the DNP Project.

ACTIVITIES

Use this tool to perform a Hazard Vulnerability Assessment for your partnering organization. Detailed instructions are available on the website.

https://www.calhospitalprepare.org/hazard-vulnerability-analysis

What emergencies could occur that might impact your DNP Project?

What contingency plans are in place to address these issues?

NEXT STEPS

- Discuss emergency planning with your DNP faculty.
- Continue to develop your skills in addressing safety and emergency preparedness.

REFERENCES AND RESOURCES

American Association of Colleges of Nursing. (2021). *The essentials: Core competencies for professional nursing education*. https://www.aacnnursing.org/Education-Resources/AACN-Essentials

Department of Homeland Security, FEMA. (2018). *Threat and hazard identification risk assessment and stakeholder preparedness review guide*. https://www.fema.gov/sites/default/files/2020-07/threat-hazard-identification-risk-assessment-stakeholder-preparedness-review-guide.pdf

FEMA. (2018). *Mission areas and core capabilities*. https://www.fema.gov/emergency-managers/national-preparedness/mission-core-capabilities

Healthy People 2030. (n.d.). *Emergency preparedness*. https://health.gov/healthypeople/objectives-and-data/browse-objectives/emergency-preparedness

Kaiser Permanente. (2021). *Hazard vulnerability assessment tool*. https://www.calhospitalprepare.org/hazard-vulnerability-analysis

LESSON 9.10

JUST CULTURE AND THE DNP PROJECT

BACKGROUND

Just culture describes an environment in which individuals feel empowered to report concerns, errors, and opportunities to improve without fear of inappropriate repercussions. As a component of the DNP Project, you should consider the impact the organizational culture will have on your results. Developing scenarios for discussion may be a worthy activity for DNP experience hours to promote learning and comprehension.

LEARNING OBJECTIVES

- Define concepts of just culture.
- List potential situations that might arise related to the DNP Project.

ACTIVITIES

Review the key concept related to just culture and its definition. Relate it to your DNP Project. Provide a rationale to support the appropriate response. An example is done for you.

CONCEPT	DEFINITION	HOW COULD IT RELATE TO YOUR DNP PROJECT?	APPROPRIATE RESPONSE AND RATIONALE
Human Error	Should have done something besides what they did.	A provider could make a prescribing mistake	The system for medication error would be triggered as soon as identified; Incident Report filed
Negligence	Failure to take expected care in a given situation.		
Intentional Rule Violation	Ignoring a rule on purpose.		
Recklessness	Disregarding a substantial risk.		

NEXT STEPS

- Discuss just culture further with your faculty and preceptor.

REFERENCE AND RESOURCE

AORN. (2023). *Just culture scenarios.* https://www.aorn.org/docs/default-source/aorn/toolkits/just-culture/just-culture-scenarios.pdf?sfvrsn=49c63c84

LESSON 9.11

INCLUSION OF INTERPROFESSIONAL INTERACTIONS

BACKGROUND

The DNP experience hours will vary. As a result, students may not have consistent opportunities in the clinical setting. Faculty and DNP students should design a consistent interprofessional experience to ensure validation of competency. In this lesson, consider activities that every DNP student could engage in to have interprofessional interactions. At a minimum, we recommend conducting an interprofessional interview.

LEARNING OBJECTIVES

ACTIVITIES

Make a list of other health professionals who might provide expert insight into your DNP Project. Identify a willing participant for a short interview. In preparation for the interview, make a list of open-ended questions to guide your conversation.

Professional:

Interview Questions:

1.
2.
3.
4.
5.

NEXT STEPS

- Incorporate their perspective into the DNP Project and share your findings with others.

REFERENCE AND RESOURCE

Cowan, L., Hartjes, T., & Munro, S. (2019). A model of successful DNP and PhD collaboration. *Journal of the American Association of Nurse Practitioners, 31*(2), 116–123.

CHAPTER SUMMARY

Here's what former DNP students have shared about their DNP practice experiences:

"Besides my DNP Project (on a different topic), I spent time in an employer-owned, on-site primary care clinic. It provided care to employees and covered dependents. I led the evaluation of their health indicators (BP, A1c, lipid profile, etc.) for an entire year. The model was so successful the owner was invited to present the model at the Centers for Disease Control Prevention in Atlanta, Georgia. I had the opportunity to be a part of the presentation and the round-table discussion at the CDC."

—Margaret Zoellers, DNP

"My goal was to offer a support group to Jewish women who have experienced pregnancy loss. To learn more, I attended several support groups on pregnancy loss in other areas of the state. Some were focused to the general population and others were specifically for Jewish women of all levels of observance (my population of interest). Although that information was not in my DNP paper, attending those meetings helped me design my intervention."

—Martha DeCrise, DNP

"Besides implementing my project, I spent a lot of time talking with the staff about the project and getting their feedback. I had regular meetings, attended a tobacco cessation training course for providers, and attended other conferences/seminars to get up to date on changes in the healthcare field (related to tobacco abuse/misuse)."

—Michelle Santoro, DNP

"I spent quite a bit of time in a clinic for pregnant women with substance abuse issues . . . and on a unit at another agency for infants with neonatal abstinence syndrome. I also shadowed a dean of nursing at another college of nursing who also specializes in perinatal research."

—Angela Clark, DNP

"The DNP experience was divided into three phases. In the planning phase, I completed the Institute for Healthcare Improvement (IHI) Open School courses to learn about the Model for Improvement. Then I hosted a kickoff party, which consisted of one-to-one education sessions on diabetes (my topic of interest), morning huddles, and use of white boards to improve communication. I developed tools, checklists, and a sticker system for providers to better identify diabetic patients. After other work, data collection, and analysis, the project work wrapped up with a SQUIRE (Standards for QUality Improvement Reporting Excellence) paper, storyboard preparation, and presentation to the facility and stakeholders."

—Tarnia Newton, DNP

The AACN asserts that a minimum of 1,000 hours of practice beyond the BSN must be performed as part of an academic program. The DNP practice experience hours should expand beyond direct patient care to embrace learning in contexts that align with the DNP *Essentials*. As you work with your faculty to determine your plan, draw on these student examples and the content of this chapter for inspiration.

10

Finishing Strong: Project Profiles and Empowerment

Editor: Jeannie Scruggs Cory
Contributors: Molly Bradshaw, Tracy R. Vitale, Linda Shepard, and Tina C. Switzer

Lessons

Lesson 10.1 DNP Project Profile: Implementing Evidence-Based Messages

Lesson 10.2 DNP Project Profile: Use of the Institute for Healthcare Improvement Model for Improvement

Lesson 10.3 DNP Project Profile: Community-Based Projects and Population Health

Lesson 10.4 DNP Project Profile: Advocacy to Create a Body of Scholarship

Lesson 10.5 DNP Project Profile: Recovering After Your Topic Changes

Lesson 10.6 DNP Project Profile: Nursing Leadership and Competency Development

Lesson 10.7 DNP Project Profile: Program Evaluation—Population Health

Lesson 10.8 The Approach to "Negative" or "Bad" Results

Lesson 10.9 Finishing on a Note of Empowerment

OBJECTIVES

In the final chapter, a series of student projects are profiled to illustrate key concepts of the workbook. The profiles summarize the key points of the selected DNP Projects, point out lessons learned, and engage other DNP students in case study. Strategies are offered to help DNP students manage common project-related problems. This chapter and the workbook conclude with a final lesson on the concept of nursing empowerment. By the end of this chapter, you will be able to

- Review the DNP Project profiles and complete the case study questions.
- Apply the tips for success to your own DNP Project.
- Utilize strategies to address common DNP Project problems.
- Commit to a future of empowering yourself and others.

INTRODUCTION

Envision completing your DNP Project. Abraham Lincoln said, "I do the very best I know how . . . and I mean to keep doing so to the end (Wise Old Sayings, n.d.)." Ah, completing your DNP Project. Even better, the climax of the DNP program—graduation. What a moment, "Congratulations, Doctor . . . (your last name)!" Your moment. This chapter offers final content to help get you to this moment, your moment, with a strong finish.

We believe in leadership by example. Therefore, we asked for the help of recent DNP graduates. We profile key features of their real-world projects to help illustrate major concepts of the workbook. These graduates were all completing their projects after publication of the American Association of Colleges of Nursing (AACN, 2015) white paper, which clarified the recommended content of the DNP Project. These students offer their experiences in overcoming the challenges of the project and present their advice for your success.

We use their projects as inspiration to challenge you. Based on what you have learned in this workbook, we ask you to apply your knowledge. There are no right or wrong answers. But if you are leading, or plan to lead, a similar project, we give you a chance to practice the skills you have learned in your doctoral journey.

The DNP Project does not occur in a vacuum. It occurs in the context of an organization, system, and population(s) with complexities. Because it is a firsthand, real-world experience, it is only natural you will experience complications, challenges, and problems. We reserve the final lessons of this workbook to help you think through strategies to manage common DNP Project–related problems.

The DNP degree should empower you to engage in the highest levels of nursing practice. As you are empowered, you should also empower others—your colleagues, your team, and, most important, your patients. Completing the DNP Project is only the beginning of the next chapter of your nursing journey. Oprah Winfrey makes a great point by saying, "Doing your best at this moment, puts you in the best spot for the next moment" (Wise Old Sayings, n.d.) Commit to a legacy of empowering self and others in the moments to come in the future. Let's begin.

REFERENCES AND RESOURCES

American Association of Colleges of Nursing. (2015). *The doctor of nursing practice: Current issues and clarifying recommendations.* [White paper]. https://www.aacnnursing.org/Portals/42/News/White-Papers/DNP-Implementation-TF-Report-8-15.pdf

Wise Old Sayings. (n.d.). *Finishing strong sayings and quotes.* http://www.wiseoldsayings.com/finishing-strong-quotes/

LESSON 10.1

DNP PROJECT PROFILE: IMPLEMENTING EVIDENCE-BASED MESSAGES

Contributing DNP Student: Angela Wood

BACKGROUND

Motivational interviewing (MI) is a common technique utilized to improve communication in DNP Projects. This project was selected because it demonstrates the use of MI for a practice change to deliver an evidence-based message, the 5-2-1-0 message. The project adds value to the current delivery of care using evidence to address factors that contribute to pediatric obesity. In addition to validated instruments, there are clear health indicators for benchmarking patient outcomes.

PROJECT PROFILE

Student: Angela Wood

Project title: "Motivational Interviewing in Primary Care to Improve Lifestyle Choices for School-Age Children" (Supplement 10.1, the full project write-up by Angela Wood, is available via Springer Publishing Connect™. Access the supplement via connect.springerpub.com/content/book/978-0-8261-7484-0/chapter/ch10 and select the "Show additional chapter resources" button.)

Problem: Obesity is becoming an epidemic in the pediatric population. Primary care providers are in an ideal position to intervene; however, they may not approach counseling in an evidence-based way using a standardized message.

Purpose statement: The purpose of the DNP Project was to change practice to utilize MI and the 5-2-1-0 message to improve delivery of information during well-child examinations. The purpose of this lesson is to use this DNP Project as a case study in which to apply your project management and leadership skills.

Implementation framework: Model for Improvement ("Plan, Do, Study, Act" or PDSA).

Intervention population: Providers and parents/guardians of patients.

Impact population: Obese children aged 4 to 12 years scheduled for well-child examinations.

Methodology:

1. Develop = Train providers in use of 5-2-1-0, MI, and process for project
2. Implement = Evidence-based message (5-2-1-0) using MI
   a. Procedure:
      I. Consent
      II. Well-child examination with MI and 5-2-1-0 message introduced at end of visit

III. 5-2-1-0 materials given, demographic survey, Family Nutrition and Physical Activity (FNPA) completed, Readiness Ruler completed, and information given to principal investigator (PI) in a sealed, numbered envelope; a 1-month follow-up was scheduled
IV. Made a 2-week follow-up phone call to reinforce information and remind of appointment
V. A 1-month follow-up appointment; FNPA and Readiness Ruler administered
3. Evaluate
    a. Describe the impact population
        I. Instrument: Self-developed demographic survey
    b. Outcome 1: Behavior modification related to nutrition and activity
        I. Instrument: The FNPA screening tool
    c. Outcome 2: Effectiveness of MI
        I. Instrument: Readiness Ruler from the *Keep Me Healthy Toolkit*

LEARNING OBJECTIVES

- Become inspired by other students.
- Apply project management and leadership skills.
- Transfer lessons learned and advice from DNP students to your DNP Project.

ACTIVITIES

Part 1: There is clear evidence on the benefit of using both MI and the 5-2-1-0 message in clinical practice. The key is how to translate that information and actually get the providers to use it in practice. Student needs must align with agency needs.

"I identified the practice gap of this clinical agency with the help of the stakeholders (leadership, providers, and staff). It's important to assess and meet the needs of the agency to improve patient outcomes. Personal interests may not align with the needs of the agency." —Angela Wood

In your project, how will you assess agency needs and align them with your needs?

_____

_____

_____

_____

"If I could change anything in hindsight, I wish I had involved the agency earlier. Their perspective of the problem may have influenced my work in the early DNP courses and prevented my project from changing focus to better align with their needs." —Angela Wood

☑️ **Part 2: Obesity is an epidemic for all ages. Benchmarking is a quality-improvement technique used to help measure patient outcomes. In regard to benchmarking health outcomes of patients, list some indicators (direct and indirect) of obesity that are improving or being impacted.**

"Since the intervention was performed at the well-child exam, we routinely document certain indicators such as height, weight, BMI (body mass index), and blood pressure. Those are certainly direct measures. We can also track the number of patients/families who return for follow-up visits using the electronic health record to show, in a more indirect way, that we are making an effort to impact obesity." —Angela Wood

List the potential indicators, or data points, that are related to your DNP Project outcomes.

_____
_____
_____
_____
_____

NEXT STEPS

- Assess the needs of your partnering agency early to better align them with your needs.
- Determine what information is routinely collected that might measure the impact of your project outcomes, directly or indirectly.

REFERENCES AND RESOURCES

Wood, A. (2017, November). *Motivational interviewing in primary care to improve lifestyle choices for school aged children. Paper presented for the degree of Doctor of Nursing Practice at.* Eastern Kentucky University.

Wood, A. (2018, April). *Motivational interviewing in primary care to improve lifestyle choices for school aged children.* Poster session presented at the 3rd Annual College of Health Sciences Scholars Day. Eastern Kentucky University.

RELATED TEXTBOOKS

Sylvia, M. L., & Terhaar, M. F. (2018). *Clinical analytics and data management for the DNP.* Springer Publishing Company.

Chapter 16: Ongoing Monitoring, Benchmarks, pages 291–307

White, K. M., Dudley-Brown, S., & Terhaar, M. F (Eds.). (2020). *Translation of evidence into nursing and healthcare* (3rd ed.). Springer Publishing Company.

Chapter 1: Evidence-Based Practice

Chapter 4: Translation of Evidence to Improve Clinical Outcomes

Chapter 9: Project Planning and the Work of Translation

Chapter 13: Interprofessional Collaboration and Practice for Translation

LESSON 10.2

DNP PROJECT PROFILE: USE OF THE INSTITUTE FOR HEALTHCARE IMPROVEMENT MODEL FOR IMPROVEMENT

Contributing DNP Student: Tarnia Newton

BACKGROUND

The Institute for Healthcare Improvement (IHI, 2019a) Model for Improvement is more commonly known as the "Plan, Do, Study, Act" or "PDSA" cycle. The goal of this model is to accelerate improvement by making and testing small changes to allow for greater implementation over time. These rapid cycles foster more immediate results and can be adjusted to meet real-world time frames (IHI, 2019a). As mentioned in a previous lesson, we recommend completing the IHI Open School Online Courses and consider utilization of the free tools available.

In this lesson, we examine a DNP Project based on use of the Model for Improvement. The student completed the IHI training mentioned and then applied it to improve care for diabetic patients in the clinical setting. There were four rapid PDSA cycles completed in the context of one DNP Project. Keep in mind that many institutional review boards (IRBs) consider quality improvement (QI) an exempt activity.

LEARNING OBJECTIVES

- Appreciate that multiple tests of change can occur in the context of a DNP Project.
- Practice drafting plans for multiple tests of change.
- Envision the potential use of the Model for Improvement in your DNP Project and beyond in future practice.

ACTIVITIES

Use this DNP Project as an exemplar to draft a plan for multiple PDSA cycles.

Student: Tarnia Newton

Project title: "Implementing a Patient-Centered Approach to Standardization of Diabetes Care in a Nurse Practitioner-Led Clinic" (Supplement 10.2, the full project write-up by Tarnia Newton, is available via Springer Publishing Connect™. Access the supplement via connect.springerpub.com/content/book/978-0-8261-7484-0/chapter/ch10 and select the "Show additional chapter resources" button.)

"The purpose of this project was to improve patient outcomes with diabetes care utilizing the *American Diabetes Association Standards of Medical Care in Diabetes* as a map for creating a plan for improvement. An initial audit based on the key elements of the guideline was conducted to assess compliance. In this population, 75% of patients had HgA1c greater than 8 mg/dL and most patients were missing preventative care measures. My goal was to improve the percentage of diabetic patients receiving standardized, appropriate diabetic care according to the ADA guidelines to 90%." —Tarnia Newton

"I would say my initial predictions were naive and I did not understand the giant task in front of me. The QI project designed consisted of four rapid plan-do-study-act (PDSA) cycles over 90 days. Each PDSA cycle was approached with tests of change and categorized into team and patient engagement as well as two process changes: (1) Diabetic Care Measures Checklist (DCMC) and (2) a preventative care referral. Each cycle was modified and implemented every 2 weeks based on team, patient feedback, and data findings. Technically running four QI projects simultaneously" (see Figure 10.1 and Table 10.1). —Tarnia Newton

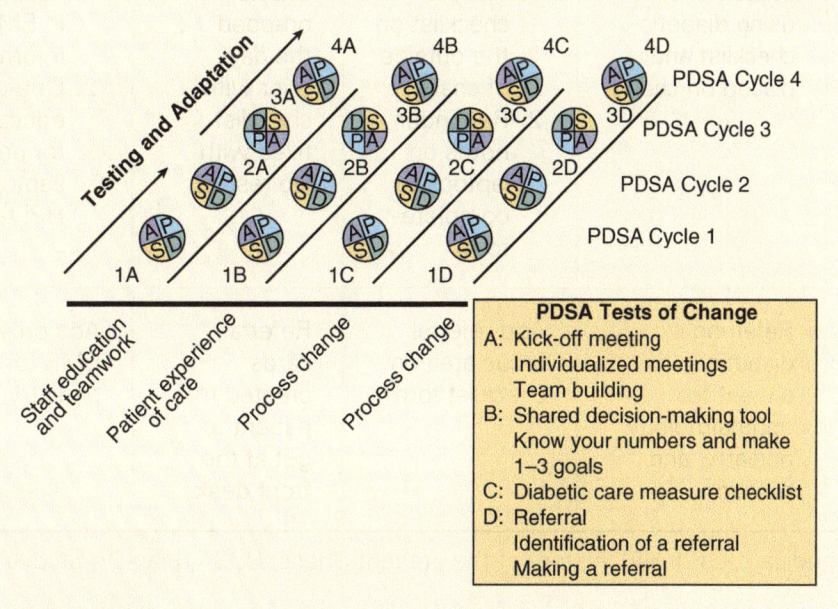

PDSA Tests of Change
A: Kick-off meeting
 Individualized meetings
 Team building
B: Shared decision-making tool
 Know your numbers and make 1–3 goals
C: Diabetic care measure checklist
D: Referral
 Identification of a referral
 Making a referral

Figure 10.1 DNP Project rapid cycle Plan-Do-Study-Act ramps. PDSA, Plan, Do, Study, Act.
Source: Reproduced with permission from Langley, G. J., Moen, R. D., Nolan, K. M., Nolan, T. W., Norman, C. L., & Provost, L. P. (2009). *The improvement guide: A practical approach to enhancing organizational performance* (2nd ed.). Jossey-Bass.

Table 10.1 Plan-Do-Study-Act Cycles and Interventions

FOCUS	PDSA #1	PDSA #2	PDSA #3	PDSA #4
Team engagement	1. Weekly team meeting 2. Implement team on diabetes teaching confidence survey	1. Add end-of PDSA-cycle meetings 2. One-on-one educational sessions with team	Initiated 10-minute morning huddles to motivate and reinforce QI	Implement a huddle white board to assist the organic engagement for the team to discuss diabetic patients for the day
Patient engagement	Patient engagement forms placed on charts for use	Creation and placement of posters in patient areas to empower diabetic patients to complete engagement forms	Engagement form prefilled with patient lab numbers	Add additional information for patients to support diabetic goals

(continued)

Table 10.1 Plan-Do-Study-Act Cycles and Interventions *(Continued)*

FOCUS	PDSA #1	PDSA #2	PDSA #3	PDSA #4
Diabetic care measure checklist	Implement using diabetic checklist and placed on chart	1. Placed checklist on the outside of chart 2. Reminder notes on laptops to complete form	Charts prepped the day prior with checklist filled with lab results	1. Create HPI template in EMR for checklist information 2. One-on-one educational session for providers to capture checklist in HPI template
Preventative care referral	Referring diabetic patient to ophthalmology, podiatry, and nutrition	Add referral focus area on checklist form	Referral cards created for patient to get at the front desk	Add provider profile in EMR for ophthalmology, podiatry, and nutrition

EMR, electronic medical record; HPI, history of the present illness; PDSA, Plan-Do-Study-Act; QI, quality improvement.

☑ Use the example of this DNP Project as inspiration. In the context of your DNP Project, if the Model for Improvement is used, how might multiple cycles fit together and build on one another? Start with the four prompts given in Figure 10.2.

Cycle on Team Engagement:

Cycle on Patient Engagement:

Cycle on Process Change 1:

Cycle on Process Change 2:

"The DNP skill set is different than anything else you might have experienced. But this process will give you the skill set required to be a change agent. Be ready to put on a new pair of glasses because you won't see healthcare the same way." —Tarnia Newton

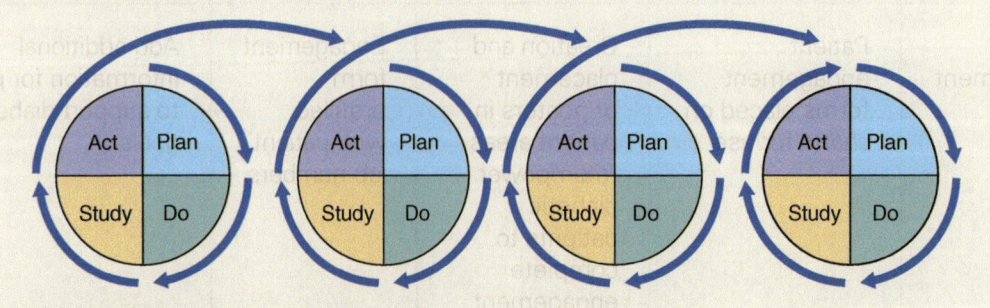

Figure 10.2 Model for Improvement.
Source: Institute for Healthcare Improvement. (2019a). How to improve. Retrieved from http://www.ihi.org/resources/Pages/HowtoImprove/default.aspx

NEXT STEPS

- Discuss your plans with your DNP team.
- Consider running multiple rapid PDSA cycles, each with a unique focus.
- Continue to utilize the Model for Improvement beyond DNP graduation.

REFERENCES AND RESOURCES

Institute for Healthcare Improvement. (2018, December). *IHI national forum on quality improvement in health care.* http://www.ihi.org/education/Conferences/Forum2017/Pages/2018-National-Forum.aspx

Institute for Healthcare Improvement. (2019a). *How to improve.* http://www.ihi.org/resources/Pages/HowtoImprove/default.aspx

Institute for Healthcare Improvement. (2019b, March). *IHI/BMJ international forum on quality and safety in healthcare.* http://internationalforum.bmj.com/

Institute for Healthcare Improvement. (2019c). *Tools.* www.ihi.org/resources/Pages/HowtoImprove/default.aspx

Institute for Healthcare Improvement. (2019d). *Open school online courses.* http://app.ihi.org/lmsspa/#/6cb1c614-884b-43ef-9abd-d90849f183d4

Langley, G. J., Moen, R. D., Nolan, K. M., Nolan, T. W., Norman, C. L., & Provost, L. P. (2009). *The improvement guide: A practical approach to enhancing organizational performance* (2nd ed.). Jossey-Bass.

Western Institute of Nursing National Conference. (2019a, April). *Improving diabetes care with TEAM engagement: A QI project (podium).* https://www.winursing.org/2019-researchconference/

Western Institute of Nursing National Conference. (2019b, April). *Improving diabetes care in a nurse-practitioner-led clinic: A QI project (poster).* https://www.winursing.org/2019-researchconference/

RELATED TEXTBOOKS

Christenbery, T (Ed.). (2018). *Evidence-based practice in nursing.* Springer Publishing Company.
   Chapter 14: Quality Improvement Processes and Evidence-Based Practice

Hickey, J. V., & Brosnan, C. A (Eds.). (2017). *Evaluation of health care quality for DNPs* (2nd ed.). Springer Publishing Company.
   Chapter 8: Quality Improvement

LESSON 10.3

DNP PROJECT PROFILE: COMMUNITY-BASED PROJECTS AND POPULATION HEALTH

Contributing DNP Student: Martha De Crisce

BACKGROUND

"Population health" is classically defined as the health outcomes of a group of individuals (Kindig & Stoddart, 2003). The American Association of Colleges of Nursing (AACN, 2015) recommends that a DNP Project has a population focus. Remember that populations exist in various places and healthcare is not always delivered in traditional clinic-based settings or hospitals. Where does your population of interest exist?

Providing healthcare to populations in a community-based setting is a feasible context for a DNP Project. The DNP Project profiled in this lesson embodies population health, evidence-based practice, engagement of community stakeholders, and collaboration with both healthcare colleagues and religious leaders. It was developed using the Centers for Disease Control and Prevention's (CDC) framework for program evaluation.

LEARNING OBJECTIVES

- Determine the importance of a "needs survey" for your DNP Project.
- Identify experts who may contribute to intervention development.
- Relate the CDC's framework for program evaluation to your current and future practice (Figure 10.3).

PROJECT PROFILE

Student: Martha De Crisce

Project title: "Addressing Pregnancy Loss Among Jewish Women" (Supplement 10.3, the full project write-up by Martha De Crisce, is available via Springer Publishing Connect™. Access the supplement via connect.springerpub.com/content/book/978-0-8261-7484-0/chapter/ch10 and select the "Show additional chapter resources" button.)

Problem: Orthodox Jewish women were lacking access to culturally appropriate resources after experiencing pregnancy loss. The current literature describes evidence for support after pregnancy loss, but it was not customized to the target population.

Purpose statement: The purpose of this DNP Project was to develop, implement, and evaluate a culturally appropriate, evidence-based support group for Orthodox Jewish women who have experienced pregnancy loss.

"My top three challenges for this project were:

1. Lack of population-specific, evidence-based literature
2. Lack of community support
3. Fear of stigma associated with pregnancy loss among the targeted population."

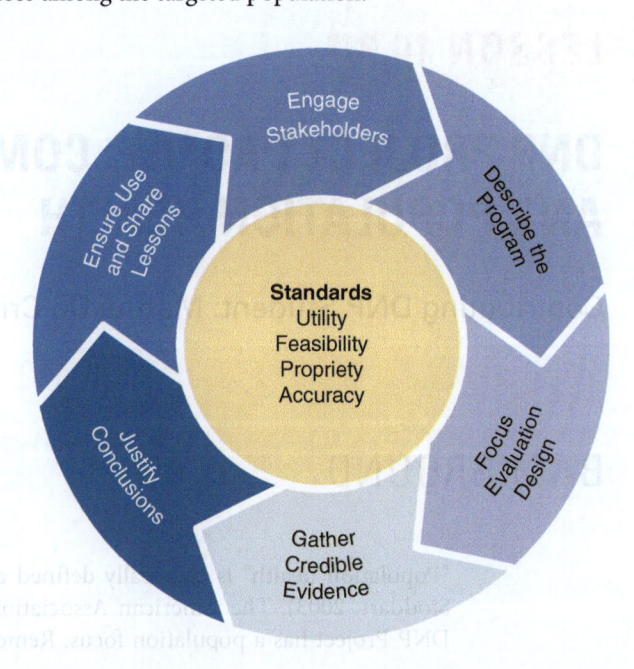

Figure 10.3 Centers for Disease Control and Prevention framework for program evaluation.
Source: Centers for Disease Control and Prevention. (1999). Framework for program evaluation in public health. *Morbidity and Mortality Weekly Report, 48*(RR-11).

"There was not much that I could do about the literature, but I could gather suggestions from the literature on pregnancy loss in other populations. There were common themes about how they perceived their loss and dealt with their emotions."

"I used this evidence to create a needs survey. It was very important for me to document the needs of my population to support the importance of my project. I used the results of the survey to design my support group. The local YM–YWHA, or Jewish Community Center, was willing to host my project. Because many Jewish women from my community were members, the center allowed me to send the survey out via its mailing list. The needs survey captured important data to present to my stakeholders." — Martha De Crisce

ACTIVITIES

Reflecting on this DNP Project, complete these activities:

Q: Should a needs survey be conducted to assess your target population? Write your thoughts here to share with your DNP team.

- What are key findings in the literature that need to be affirmed or denied?
- Are there logical questions you need to ask?

The DNP experience hours can be critical to the development of the project intervention. "Before implementing my project, I attended several support groups for pregnancy loss. Some were for my target population and some were not, but it helped me get a sense of what worked and what didn't." Martha De Crisce

Q: Could you attend similar events related to your DNP Project? Explore possible events and list them here:

Community leaders, experts, and stakeholders can help operationalize the DNP Project.

"I engaged the support of the local rabbi(s). They saw a need and were open to embracing a support group. The sensitive, religious nature of this topic and this population made their input critical. I was also supported by a psychiatrist, who was instrumental in developing the content of each session for the support group. I did undergo full IRB review since my target population was a vulnerable population." —Martha De Crisce

Q: Are there leaders, experts, or stakeholders who could/should contribute to your DNP Project? Write your notes here, listing names and possible contributions.

Q: Are you involved in a community-based program (project related or otherwise) that would benefit from improved evaluation? How can you use your DNP skills to be instrumental in evaluating the program's success? Write your notes here.

NEXT STEPS

- "Focus on a problem you are passionate about. It would be difficult to put forth so much hard work and effort toward a topic/problem that has little meaning to you."
- "Find a team that supports your vision that has open-minded members. A good team is one that supports your project and makes good recommendations to improve it." —Martha De Crisce

REFERENCES AND RESOURCES

American Association of Colleges of Nursing. (2015). *The doctor of nursing practice: Current issues and clarifying recommendations. [White paper].* https://www.aacnnursing.org/Portals/42/News/White-Papers/DNP-Implementation-TF-Report-8-15.pdf

Centers for Disease Control and Prevention. (1999). Framework for program evaluation in public health. *Morbidity and Mortality Weekly Report, 48*(RR-11).

Centers for Disease Control and Prevention. (2019). *Framework for program evaluation.* https://www.cdc.gov/eval/framework/index.htm

De Crisce, M. (2018, May). Addressing pregnancy loss among Jewish women.*Poster session presented at the Orthodox Jewish Nurses Association Annual Conference.* https://jewishnurses.org/past-conferences/conference/

Kindig, D., & Stoddart, G. (2003). What is population health? *American Journal of Public Health, 93*(3), 380–383.

RELATED TEXTBOOK

Curley, A. L., & Vitale, P. A. (2016). *Population-based nursing.* Springer Publishing Company.
  Chapter 2: Identifying Outcomes
  Chapter 10: Challenges in Program Implementation

LESSON 10.4

DNP PROJECT PROFILE: ADVOCACY TO CREATE A BODY OF SCHOLARSHIP

Contributing DNP Student: Aleksandra Novik

BACKGROUND

The DNP Project profiled in this lesson demonstrates a practice change in a small, private primary care office that eventually made an impact at the state and national levels by engaging in advocacy. Advocacy was accomplished by a series of presentations, contact with local legislators, and publication of the project on a public website. These DNP experiences generated interest that eventually caught the attention of the governor's office and Dr. Margaret Fitzgerald.

The American Association of Colleges of Nursing (AACN, 2015) advocates for use of the DNP Project as a platform for future scholarship. We add that the DNP experience also provides an opportunity to create a body of scholarship.

PROJECT PROFILE

Student: Aleksandra Novik

Project title: "Use of Controlled Dangerous Substance Tools by Advanced Practice Nurses in the State of New Jersey" (Supplements 10.4 and 10.5, the full project write-up by Aleksandra Novik, are available via Springer Publishing Connect™. Access the supplement via connect.springerpub.com/content/book/978-0-8261-7484-0/chapter/ch10 and select the "Show additional chapter resources" button.)

Problem: Nurse practitioners (NPs) and other providers prescribing opioids may not fully utilize available resources or best evidence. In a small, private practice, an NP requested development of a better form to use when signing controlled substance contracts with patients. Also, at the time, there was a new requirement to inform patients of local places to drop off unused prescription drugs, but many providers were unaware of the resource.

The purpose of this DNP Project was to close this practice gap by

- Creating an evidence-based controlled substance agreement form meeting the requirements of the state and at the appropriate level of health literacy.
- Vetting the form through practicing NPs and implementing it into practice.
- Developing an advocacy initiative to utilize state resources, such as the controlled substance monitoring program and prescription drop-off locations.

Purpose statement: The purpose of this lesson is to demonstrate the impact of advocacy as a strategy to affect both organizational and public policy as well as build a body of scholarship.

LEARNING OBJECTIVES

- Discuss opportunities to scale DNP Projects with advocacy.
- Develop a plan to create multiple presentations and a body of DNP scholarship.

ACTIVITIES

When DNP Projects occur in small settings, there is often concern that the practice change is "not enough" for doctoral work. Advocating for best practices by offering tools is a way to scale the DNP Project and impact policy. Review the components of this project, listed on the left. Next to each activity, identify and discuss opportunities related to your DNP Project.

ADVOCACY EXAMPLE	ADVOCACY OPPORTUNITY FOR YOUR DNP PROJECT
Offer evidence-based tools via a website platform. Visit this project's website at https://aleksandranovik.wixsite.com/cdsmonitoringtools	
Foster local engagement of patients by sharing information on controlled substances at a local health fair.	

(continued)

ADVOCACY EXAMPLE	ADVOCACY OPPORTUNITY FOR YOUR DNP PROJECT
Gain statewide engagement of nursing professionals by using poster presentation regarding state policy at prescription drop-off points.	
Encourage national engagement of NPs via poster presentation regarding the outcome of the project survey and the evidence-based controlled substance agreement.	
Schedule meeting with local legislators' offices to share evidence-based tools related to public policies.	

☑ Pearls and Evidence of Advocacy Success

"Participate in conferences and presentations as much as possible at all levels. Pick different components of your work to focus on at each presentation so that the presentations are not identical. This provides an opportunity to become known as a topic expert and leads to new opportunities. For example, Dr. Margaret Fitzgerald approached me at my poster at the American Association of Nurse Practitioners national conference and invited me to contribute to her monthly newsletter!" — Aleksandra Novik

"I was invited to speak at a conference on opioids at Drew University. A member of the governor's office was in attendance and approached me afterward to share my work with a state task force on opioid prescribing policies. Having my tool on a website platform made sharing the work easy. The fact that I vetted the form and surveyed nurse practitioners to understand their habits regarding controlled substances provided data and credibility to my work." — Aleksandra Novik

NEXT STEPS

- "Learn about what your DNP colleagues are doing and identify opportunities to work together. For example, I partnered with a DNP student to review my tool for components of health literacy. If you develop tools to use with patients, ensure they are both evidence based and health literacy appropriate." — Aleksandra Novik
- "Prior to DNP graduation, I completed three poster presentations and two podium presentations. Work with faculty who are both knowledgeable but also vested in the subject matter. I learned about the importance of sharing the changes I make in my clinical practice with others. I encourage you to do the same." — Aleksandra Novik

REFERENCES AND RESOURCES

American Association of Colleges of Nursing. (2015). *The doctor of nursing practice: Current issues and clarifying recommendations.* [White paper]. https://www.aacnnursing.org/Portals/42/News/White-Papers/DNP-Implementation-TF-Report-8-15.pdf

Bradshaw, M., VanWyck, K., & Novik, A. (2017, April 3). *Research to reality: Taking action in primary care to address the opioid epidemic.* Podium presentation at the Symposium on Combating Opioids and the Addiction Crisis.

Fitzgerald Health Education Associates. (2017). *Controlled dangerous substance agreement form. Newsletter*, October. 2017 https://www.fhea.com/newsletter.aspx

Novik, A. (2017). *CDS monitoring tools*. https://aleksandranovik.wixsite.com/cdsmonitoringtools/results

Novik, A., Padovano, C., & Bradshaw, M. (2016a). *NJ prescription monitoring program.* Poster presented at the Morristown Medical Center

Novik, A., Padovano, C., & Bradshaw, M. (2016b). *Project medicine drop.* Poster Presentation.Association Annual Conference.

Novik, A., Padovano, C., & Bradshaw, M. (2017). *Use of CDS agreement forms by NJ NPs.*Poster presented at the American Association of Nurse Practitioner National Conference.

RELATED TEXTBOOKS

Goudreau, K. A., & Smolenski, M. C. (2018). *Health policy and the advanced practice nurse.* Springer Publishing Company.

Grady, P. A., & Hinshaw, A. S. (2017). *Using nursing research to shape health policy.* Springer Publishing Company.

Zalon, M., & Patton, R. (2019). *Nursing making policy* (2nd ed.). Springer Publishing Company.

LESSON 10.5

DNP PROJECT PROFILE: RECOVERING AFTER YOUR TOPIC CHANGES

Student Contributor: Margaret Zoellers

BACKGROUND

The goals of the partnering agency and DNP student must be in alignment, following an agreed-upon timetable. Despite the best efforts to collaborate and/or control variables, sometimes complicated circumstances arise. The DNP student may need to change topics and/or change the location of the DNP Project as a result.

LEARNING OBJECTIVES

- Review the DNP Project profile.
- Remember to utilize the recovery questions if needed.

ACTIVITIES

Review the following DNP Project profile.

Project Profile

Student: Margaret Zoellers

Project title: "A Process Improvement for Depression Screening and Management in a University Health Clinic" (Supplement 10.6, the full project write-up by Margaret Zoellers, is available via Springer Publishing Connect™. Access the supplement via connect.springerpub.com/content/book/978-0-8261-7484-0/chapter/ch10 and select the "Show additional chapter resources" button.)

"My initial DNP Project site was awesome! An employer had established on-site primary care for employees and their dependents. I spent some time there helping them collect data on health indicators such as A1c, lipid levels, BMI, blood pressure, and so on. I was ultimately planning to implement my DNP Project there. Unfortunately, there was an unexpected health challenge for the clinic director, who had to be temporarily replaced during recovery. As a result, the employer/clinic owner felt adding a DNP Project during this period would become too difficult to manage. I had to change sites, which meant changing topics." —Margaret Zoellers

INITIAL PROJECT	FINAL PROJECT
Location: On-site, employer-sponsored health clinic Target population: Employees and dependents of the agency Problem: Identification of chronic disease indicators and improvement of population health through primary care services and lifestyle modification (Model presented to the Centers for Disease Control and Prevention [CDC])	Location: University student health clinic Target population: Students and providers involved in student health services Problem: Improving process for depression screening and treatment

Reflect on the circumstances described here and discuss the scenario with your DNP team.

- Is it appropriate to "relocate" a project from one site to another?
- What are the challenges associated with that?

In the event of unforeseen circumstances, reflect on these recovery questions:

- Is there a different organization interested in the same problem?
- Would that organization be willing to partner with the DNP student?
- What elements of the project would change if the location changes?

"A change of agency after beginning to formulate a project plan was disheartening. I lost a semester of work and time that would have provided the groundwork for my project. There was no option except to begin again with a new agency/problem. I utilized the skills from my core DNP courses to start again. Feeling overwhelmed by the unfamiliar process, I reached out to my DNP advisor often, but also peers and other qualified people for input, guidance, and encouragement." — Margaret Zoellers

Make a list of people who you can reach out to for input, guidance, and encouragement during your DNP Project process:

1.
2.
3.

As you have noticed, there have been several steps and hurdles to overcome as you plan, develop, and implement your project. Your project has likely evolved from the time you started thinking about what you would like to study. However, sometimes along the way, for a variety of reasons, the project changes. This is different from the project evolving. This may require a complete change in focus or topic. Although this may be extremely discouraging and outside your control, being equipped with strategies to recover will help you navigate this process.

Be proactive rather than reactive. Certainly, it is understandable that you may be upset about the circumstances surrounding why your project has changed, but be proactive and keep yourself moving forward. This too shall pass, and soon enough you will be well on your way with a new topic.

Be adaptable and flexible. Recognize that although you were committed to the previous project, it is now necessary to be adaptable and flexible in considering the new project topic.

Consider uncertainties that come along with a project. You have already had to adjust to different stakeholders influencing the development of the project and what that entails. That said, you will want to consider how they may contribute to any uncertainties related to your project.

Remain confident. We could argue the point that everything happens for a reason, but that may provide little consolation while you are in the thick of it and trying to start from scratch.

NEXT STEPS

- "Identify a student peer for collaboration and moral support."
- "Realize that you are likely not going to change the world with your DNP Project—but you will make a difference." — Margaret Zoellers

REFERENCE AND RESOURCE

Zoellers, M. H. (2018). *A process improvement for depression screening and management in a University Health Clinic.* Doctor of Nursing Practice Capstone Projects. 34 https://encompass.eku.edu/dnpcapstones/34

RELATED TEXTBOOK

White, K. M., Dudley-Brown, S., & Terhaar, M. F (Eds.). (2020). *Translation of evidence into nursing and healthcare* (3rd ed.). Springer Publishing Company.
Chapter 15: Best Practices in Translation: Challenges and Barriers in Translation

LESSON 10.6

DNP PROJECT PROFILE: NURSING LEADERSHIP AND COMPETENCY DEVELOPMENT

Contributing DNP Student: Linda Shepherd

BACKGROUND

Worldwide, effective nursing leadership is critical in implementing strategic objectives to drive quality patient outcomes, positive unit cultures, organizational success, and outperform external peers within a competitive environment (Asiri et al., 2016; Fennimore & Wolfe, 2011; Spiva et al., 2021). Aggressive environments have heightened the awareness and urgency in creating expansively competent, influential nurse leaders. Direct, shared observations by senior nurse leaders and mock survey results from the 2019 Joint Commission International (JCI) validated the need for further leadership development. The context of this project highlights challenges in nursing leadership and competency development in an international context.

LEARNING OBJECTIVES

- Examine real-world challenges in leadership and competency development.
- List the challenges associated with an international project.

PROJECT PROFILE

Student: Linda Shepherd

Project title: "Developing Influential Nurse Leaders: Utilizing Strengths and Styles Assessments to Create Individualized, Intentional Coaching" (available November 15, 2024, from https://commons.lib.jmu.edu/dnp202029/26/).

Context:

A north-central Virginia university and a hospital in the British West Indies (BWI) entered into a collaborative agreement in 2020. Growing competitive environments heightened awareness and urgency in creating expansively competent, influential nurse leaders in the BWI. Without formalized data to quantify or validate nurse manager strengths, leadership style, or competencies, an assessment of these items was performed and followed by an evidence-based coaching intervention.

Problem: In this international project site, there were no formalized data to quantify or validate nurse leader strengths, leadership styles, or competencies. As a result, there was an inability to meet organizational objectives, successfully navigate change, enhance nursing cultural environments, and create ongoing team accountability.

ACTIVITIES

Q: What leadership challenges/problems could be considered as potential impactful DNP projects? Make your list. Then review the answers that follow from another DNP student. Highlight similar findings.

A: "In my experience as a DNP Student, the following serve as examples of projects related to leadership and competency development." —Linda Shepard

- Nurse staffing alternatives which support work–life balance
- Working to the full extent of licensure/patient benefits
- Impact of artificial intelligence to positively affect nursing
- Nursing leadership development residency programs—are they needed and are they beneficial
- Healthy work environments
- Nursing resilience and burnout
- Retention and recognition
- Adequacy of training of healthcare workers
- Patient experience/outcomes and staffing
- Patient care reimbursement targeted at nursing care outcomes—reinvesting in nursing

Q: What challenges are involved when a DNP Project has an international focus? Make your list. Then review the answers that follow from another DNP student. Highlight similar findings.

A: "International projects are challenging! The top three challenges for this project were:

1. Multiple competing organizational priorities
2. Cultural attributes—ego and pride
3. Impact of COVID-19 aftermath" —Linda Shepard

Continue to read and discuss your observations of this student's experience.

"First, multiple competing organizational priorities were palpable throughout the enterprise, with the majority landing on nursing leadership. The organization was preparing its initial Joint Commission International (JCI) accreditation survey. The organization's JCI journey began ten years prior. However, a recent SWAT and gap analysis performed in the spring of 2022 revealed a monumental amount of work required within an abbreviated timeframe (less than eight months), with a vast amount of work to be performed by nursing managers. In addition, the organization's strategic plan focused on thirty-plus initiatives, which also required frontline leader involvement and timelines paralleling the JCI survey.

"The situation was compounded by a lack of nursing staff and complex and lengthy human resource hiring and onboarding processes, pushing nurse leaders into staffing weekly. While simultaneously requiring these leaders to oversee operations and fill in for house supervision as needed. Such requirements resulted in minimal time to focus on leadership development and nominal structures supporting development. In recognizing the need for development, multiple strategies required deployment. Such strategies included gaining support from the Chief Nursing Officer, the executive leadership team, human resources (responsible for leadership development), and nurse managers focusing on the importance of leadership development within a competitive environment, which tied to the JCI rationale for obtaining accreditation. Creative, flexible scheduling for coaching was proactively created, multiple mediums for coaching sessions were offered, and solidified dates and times mutually agreed upon for coaching sessions were sent as reminders through calendar invites. Coaching plans were built on individual strengths to fill gaps and minimize the learning curve.

"The second challenge focused on the cultural attributes of ego and pride. Pride and ego are culturally prevalent within the vastly cultured society, resulting in a lack of acknowledgment by some nurse leaders related to the gravity of the need for development. From an organizational perspective, leaders exhibited great pride in their knowledge and ability to make staff happy. Personal observations and conversations with organizational leaders originating from outside the BWI region revealed a lack of accountability of staff by leadership and a failure to address issues to not create adverse feelings among co-workers or subordinates, lending to perceived negative feelings directed toward the leader. The project would require sharing information related to gaps in leadership development and developmental coaching, which, for those who possess pride and high egos, discussing such information would be tenuous and successful with a significant level of trust between the project owner and each nurse leader. Strategies included spending multiple hours daily with nursing leadership and their teams to understand their roles and build trust. In working with the nurse leaders, other cultural sensitivities were identified and considered through emotional intelligence and cultural sensitivity. These strategies and tactics were essential to maintain trust and mutual respect while facilitating learning.

"Finally, the aftermath of COVID-19 resulted in exhaustion among nurses and nurse leaders everywhere; the BWI was no exception. The borders were closed for the previous two and a half years, and nursing leadership received no days off, per the Chief Nursing Officer. Since the island's reopening, the nurse leaders had the opportunity to engage in time off for extended periods (2-6 weeks), which created challenges from a timing perspective related to the project. These challenges required flexibility related explicitly to the coaching segment of the project. As previously described, creative scheduling and alternative coaching mediums were offered to assist in navigating this challenge. When scheduled appointments were missed, flexibility was offered through rescheduling at a time conducive to the nurse leader. Projects can quickly derail without anticipating and investigating potential challenges and proactive solutions." —Linda Shepherd

What additional thoughts and concerns do you have based on this experience?

NEXT STEPS

Here is some final advice from our DNP student contributor, Linda Shepherd:

- "Focus on a problem that has meaning to you. The journey to project completion is long, therefore one must be fueled by passion and excitement, so make sure the topic is one that you are passionate about."
- "Surround yourself with those who support you and your project. Feedback and a new perspective are always helpful."
- "Ask for help and guidance when needed. Struggling alone is no fun and only causes frustration."
- "Best of luck. Take time to care for yourselves throughout the process. You will all do great and make it to the finish line."

REFERENCES AND RESOURCES

Asiri, S. A., Rohrer, W. W., Al-Surimi, K., Da'ar, O. O., & Ahmed, A. (2016). The association of leadership styles and empowerment with nurses' organizational commitment in an acute health care setting: A cross-sectional study. *BMC Nurse*, *15*(38), 28–36. https://doi.org/10.1186/s12912-016-0161-7

Clifton, D. (2008). *Strength based leadership*. Gallup Press.

Fennimore, L., & Wolf, G. (2011). Nurse manager leadership development. *The Journal of Nursing Administration*, *41*(5), 204–210. https://doi.org/10.1097/NNA.0b013e3182171aff

Paterson, K., Henderson, A., & Burmeister, E. (2015). The impact of a leadership development program on nurses' self-perceived leadership capability. *Journal of Nursing Management*, *23*(8), 1086–1093. https://doi.org/10.1111/jonm.12257

Spiva, L., Hedenstrom, L., Ballard, N., Buitrago, P., Davis, S., Hogue, V., Box, M., Taasoobshirazi, G., & Case-Wirth, J. (2021). Nurse leader training and strength-based coaching. *Nursing Management*, *52*(10), 42–50.

Zuberbuhler, M., Salanova, M., & Martinez, I. (2020). Coached-based leadership intervention program: A controlled trial study. *Frontiers in Psychology*, *12*(2). https://doi.org/10.3389/fpsyg.2019.03066

LESSON 10.7

DNP PROJECT PROFILE: PROGRAM EVALUATION—POPULATION HEALTH

Contributing DNP Student: Tina C. Switzer

BACKGROUND AND PROBLEM

Program evaluation is a framework that could be used to guide the development, implementation, and evaluation of a DNP Project. In this lesson, you will examine a student who completed a project using this type of project design.

LEARNING OBJECTIVES

- Explore program evaluation as a potential DNP project.
- Compare program evaluation frameworks utilized in DNP Projects

PROJECT PROFILE

Student: Tina C. Switzer

Project title: "Registered Nurse-Led Annual Wellness Visits in Rural Health Clinics: A Program Evaluation of a New Role" (Supplement 10.7, the full project write-up by Tina Switzer, is available via Springer Publishing Connect™. Access the supplement via connect.springerpub.com/content/book/978-0-8261-7484-0/chapter/ch10 and select the "Show additional chapter resources" button.)

Context:

In 2019, a Health Resources Services Administration (HRSA) Grant–sponsored program hired two RNs to train for and demonstrate full-scope primary care nursing roles. They were introduced to and immersed in five rural health clinics (RHCs) in a rural Virginia county to help manage patient care needs and expand access for both preventive and chronic illness care. The RNs created population health initiatives, managed care transitions and complex care needs, and offered free patient education and counseling visits. The RNs also initiated a new model of shared provider encounters, including annual wellness visits (AWVs). A literature search demonstrated that the role creation and impact of RN interventions specifically in RHCs has not been comprehensively explored; therefore, a program evaluation of this role through the lens of the AWV was conducted to determine if there were positive patient and clinic impacts as well as reveal opportunities for program improvement (Gielen & Eileen, 1996).

ACTIVITIES

Q: What frameworks might be used to guide a Program Evaluation DNP Project? Review the Centers for Disease Control and Prevention (CDC) framework and compare it to the framework utilized by the DNP student.

- Centers for Disease Control and Prevention, Framework for Program Evaluation.
  Visit: https://www.cdc.gov/evaluation/index.*htm*

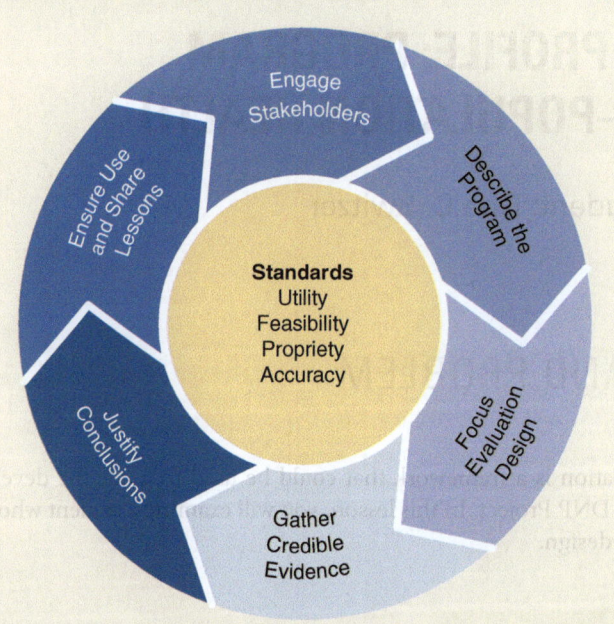

What do you like and dislike about this framework? Make a list.

I LIKE . . .	I DISLIKE . . .

- PRECEDE/PROCEED Model
  Visit: https://ctb.ku.edu/en/table-contents/overview/other-models-promoting-community-health-and-development/preceder-proceder/main

[PRECEDE-PROCEED Model diagram]

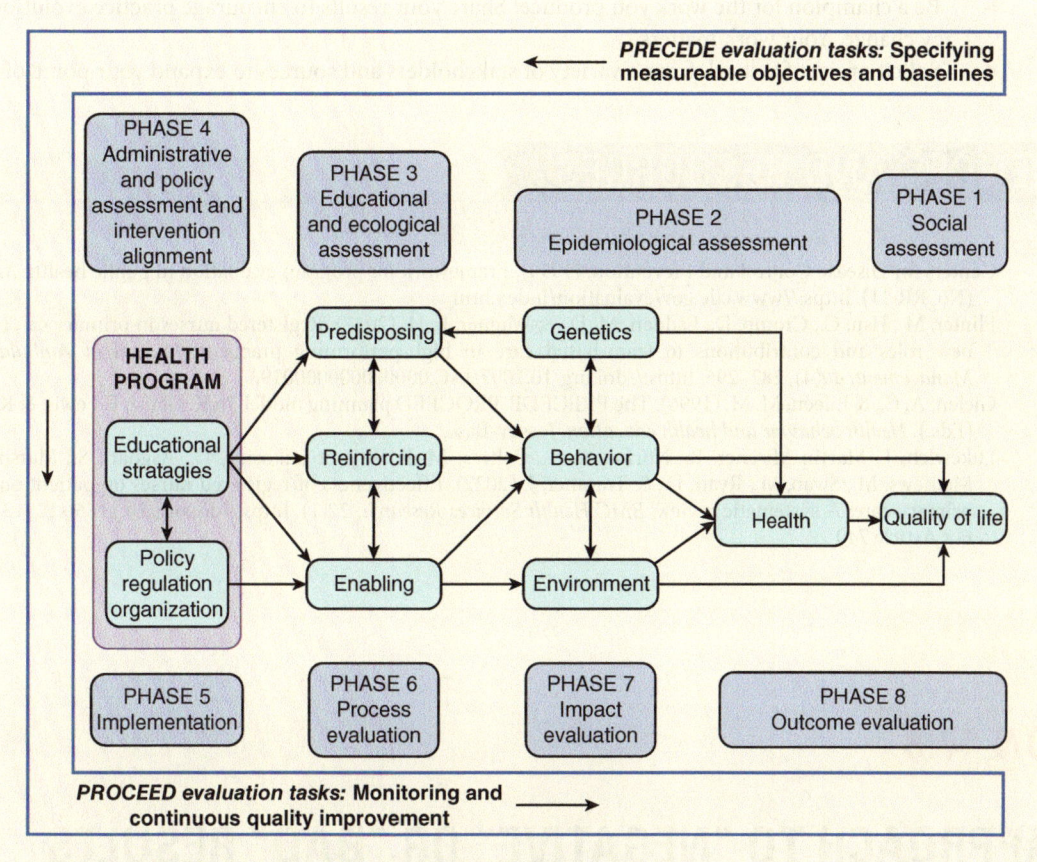

PRECEDE evaluation tasks: Specifying measurable objectives and baselines

- PHASE 4: Administrative and policy assessment and intervention alignment
- PHASE 3: Educational and ecological assessment
- PHASE 2: Epidemiological assessment
- PHASE 1: Social assessment

HEALTH PROGRAM: Educational strategies; Policy regulation organization

Predisposing → Behavior; Reinforcing → Behavior; Enabling → Environment; Genetics → Behavior; Behavior → Health; Environment → Health; Health → Quality of life

- PHASE 5: Implementation
- PHASE 6: Process evaluation
- PHASE 7: Impact evaluation
- PHASE 8: Outcome evaluation

PROCEED evaluation tasks: Monitoring and continuous quality improvement

What do you like and dislike about this framework? Make a list.

I LIKE . . .	I DISLIKE . . .

"RN roles in primary care settings (and most certainly in Rural Health Clinics) are in great need of thorough program evaluation. New models of care which are RN-centric including Chronic Care Management, transitional support, population health interventions (vaccination initiatives, hypertension clinics, diabetes education, advance directive completion) are excellent opportunities for evaluation of new models of care to determine overall impact for possible replication in similar settings.

The measures were determined by the direct screening and wellness/prevention interventions that were provided by the RNs as recommended by the Centers for Medicare and Medicaid Services for Annual Wellness Visits. The literature suggested that there is evidence to support that AWVs increase screening completions and decreased hospital encounter rates after the AWV. The intent was to determine if similar outcomes could be demonstrated in Rural Health Clinics where RN role impact has not been clearly explored. Furthermore, the fiscal sustainability of primary care RN roles has not been clearly demonstrated in the overall literature so this was an important domain to explore to ensure the future of this important resource." —Tina C. Switzer

NEXT STEPS

Here is some final advice from our DNP student contributor, Tina C. Switzer:

- "Look at meaningful work or interventions that you are passionate about but try to keep the scope of your project at a manageable and focused level to be able to produce a comprehensive project that is not muddled or difficult to replicate or build upon. Sometimes less is more!"

- "Be a champion for the work you produce! Share your results to encourage practice evolution or policy change. Your work matters."
- "Solicit project feedback from a variety of stakeholders and sources to expand your point-of-view."

REFERENCES AND RESOURCES

Centers for Disease Control and Prevention. (1999). Framework for program evaluation in public health. *MMWR*. 48 (No. RR-11). https://www.cdc.gov/evaluation/index.htm

Flinter, M., Hsu, C., Cromp, D., Ladden, M. D., & Wagner, E. H. (2017). Registered nurses in primary care: Emerging new roles and contributions to team-based care in high-performing practices. *Journal of Ambulatory Care Management*, 40(4), 287–296. https://doi.org/10.1097/JAC.0000000000000193

Gielen, A. C., & Eileen, M. M. (1996). The PRECEDE-PROCEED planning model. In K. Glanz, F. Lewis, & K. B. Rimer (Eds.), *Health behavior and health education*. Jossey-Bass.

Lukewich, J., Martin-Misener, R., Norful, A. A., Poitras, M.-E., Bryant-Lukosius, D., Asghari, S., Marshall, E. G., Mathews, M., Swab, M., Ryan, D., & Tranmer, J. (2022). Effectiveness of registered nurses on patient outcomes in primary care: A systematic review. *BMC Health Services Research*, 22(1). https://doi.org/10.1186/s12913-022-07866-x Article 740

LESSON 10.8

THE APPROACH TO "NEGATIVE" OR "BAD" RESULTS

BACKGROUND

It is helpful to remember that the DNP Project is a learning experience. It is an opportunity to develop, implement, and evaluate practice improvements with the help and support of your DNP team. The list that follows contains some frequently asked questions regarding negative or bad results.

LEARNING OBJECTIVES

- Appreciate the importance of a "negative" or "bad" result.
- Articulate DNP Project limitations with transparency.

Q: *"What if my DNP Project does not show 'statistical' significance?"*
A: *Statistical significance* refers to the amount of certainty there is that the intervention (independent variable) caused the result. Its lack does not mean that the DNP Project is not meaningful.

Q: *"What if my DNP Project results are 'negative' or 'bad'"?*
A: Even evidence-based interventions can be unsuccessful. But that's okay! According to Dr. Irina Benenson, "If an intervention doesn't produce the outcome we want, we should consider abandoning the practice or trying a different approach." A negative result simply means that you have to do something different.

Q: *"Should I only report the good information and omit the bad?"*
A: No, report results and limitations with accuracy and transparency. As a student, you should try to consider what factors contributed to the negative result. Report things as they actually happened. Discuss the limitations of the DNP Project.

ACTIVITIES

Talk to your faculty members hypothetically about what happens if the outcome of your DNP Project is not favorable. Record the key points of the discussion here.

Expert Commentary: Tracy R. Vitale, DNP, RNC-OB, C-EFM, NE-BC

When I conducted my DNP Project, I was devastated when I completed my data analysis and found negative results. As some background, I was looking to identify how participating in a structured mentorship program impacted nurse leaders' transformational leadership practices and job satisfaction. I double- and triple-checked my results because I must have done something wrong in the analysis. Maybe I had mixed up my categories? Maybe I had clicked the wrong button? But no . . . I had negative results!

I felt defeated, disappointed, and as if all my work had been for nothing. After a long (ugly) cry, I reached out to my project chair and asked for help. He calmly talked me down and said, "Your data are your data. You can't change that. What you can do is to examine your results and consider possible reasons why that happened and speak to it." If you have negative results, use the information for your benefit and speak to what may have influenced the results. In my case, most of my sample of nurse leaders were in their mid-50s. It is likely that regardless of having participated in the structured mentoring, the two groups likely received mentoring in some capacity, at some point in their 20- to 30+-year nursing careers. My results could also have been different had I used a better project design. There are several factors (limitations) that may have been the reason for my results. The bottom line is your results are your results . . . and that's okay!

Looking back, I wish someone would have prepared me for the possibility of negative results. Perhaps then I would not have panicked like I did or worried that I would not be able to graduate. In fact, the more I talked about my results and surprised people with them, the more confidently I was able to speak to the potential whys, how I could have improved my project, or how I can use those results for future research and scholarly work. There was a benefit in having my results be what they were; I was able to use my DNP education and speak to how the results align/do not align with existing evidence. I am able to see the importance of project design and methodology impacting the quality of the DNP Project. Also, perhaps what I am most proud of is that in a time when we encourage students to work toward publishing their DNP work, I, too, was able to publish the results of my DNP Project—negative results and all!

So, although your results may be negative, you must stay positive! Learn from the experience and use the fundamentals you studied in your doctoral classes to identify and analyze why you had those results, recommend opportunities to address those factors and limitations, and keep moving forward! Remember . . . negative results do not equal failure, but rather more evidence to contribute to the greater body of knowledge. Your data matters just as much as everyone else's data, so keep your chin up and be proud of the work you have done.

NEXT STEPS

- Discuss the potential outcomes of negative results with your DNP team.
- Stay encouraged even if the results of the project are not what you expect.

RELATED TEXTBOOK

Sylvia, M. L., & Terhaar, M. F. (2019). *Clinical analytics and data management for the DNP*. Springer Publishing Company.

LESSON 10.9

FINISHING ON A NOTE OF EMPOWERMENT

BACKGROUND

The DNP Project and the DNP degree are instruments of nursing empowerment. "Empowerment" essentially means being equipped or having the ability to get things done (Christenbery, 2018). You are now equipped with essential skills to solve complex healthcare problems and lead interprofessional teams. You can develop, implement, and evaluate the impact of evidence-based solutions on patient outcomes.

LEARNING OBJECTIVES

- Describe the contribution your doctoral work has made.
- Relate the meaning of the work to elements of an empowered organization.

What do you think of when you think of empowerment? How do you empower yourself? How do you empower others?

ACTIVITIES

Consider the empowering behaviors listed in Box 10.1. Highlight the three that are most important to you.

Box 10.1 Example of Empowering Behaviors

Organizations that encourage empowerment provide the following:

- Opportunities for professional growth and development
- Stimulating and challenging work
- Opportunities to gain new work-related knowledge and skills
- Access to resources to accomplish work
- Time allotted to complete work
- Encouragement to find meaning in work
- Information needed to accomplish work
- Support from management to meet responsibilities and work activities
- Opportunities to work collaboratively with other departments and interprofessional teams
- Recognition for work well done
- Tangible recognition from organizational leadership for the work done

Source: From Christenbery, T. (Ed.). (2018). *Evidence-based practice in nursing.* Springer Publishing Company.

☑ **Based on your selections, list two ways that you will continue to foster these behaviors after graduation:**

1.

2.

☑ **Briefly describe the meaning and contribution your doctoral work has made.**

Contribution to your personal/professional growth:

Contribution to your partnering organization:

Contribution to the nursing profession:

NEXT STEP

- Empower self and others in your future endeavors.

REFERENCE AND RESOURCE

Christenbery, T (Ed.). (2018). *Evidence-based practice in nursing.* Springer Publishing Company.

RELATED TEXTBOOKS

Christenbery, T (Ed.). (2018). *Evidence-based practice in nursing.* Springer Publishing Company.
  Chapter 15: Evidence-Based Practice: A Culture of Organizational Empowerment
  Chapter 20: Evidence-Based Practice: Empowering Nurses

CHAPTER SUMMARY

Consider how far you have come since you started this journey toward the DNP. You will soon be a doctorally prepared nurse leader. You will be qualified at the highest level of nursing practice. Take a minute to look back at where you started just a short time ago. It is likely that somewhere along the way you were inspired by another nurse leader, a colleague, a faculty member, or even another student. Remember to be that source of inspiration for others in the future. It is now your moment to carry that forward and, as Mahatma Gandhi said, "be the change you wish to see in the world." We are confident that you will finish strong!

Appendix: Project Management Resources

COMMUNICATION FORM

DNP student:_____   Date:_____

Other attendees:
_____
_____

Purpose of the meeting/communication:
_____
_____

Notes:
_____
_____

Action items:
_____
_____

Timeline for completion:
_____

Next scheduled meeting:
_____

Other plans for follow-up:
_____
_____

GROUP PROJECT PLANNING FORM

The American Association of Colleges of Nursing (AACN, 2015) specifies that although group projects can be valuable, they do present some challenges, especially when it comes to evaluation/grading them. AACN (2015) also indicates that each member of a project team must successfully meet all expectations of planning, implementation, and evaluation and the work of each must be evaluated separately. Students who are completing a group DNP project should submit this form to the DNP chair for approval at the beginning of the DNP planning process.

REQUIREMENTS	STUDENT A	STUDENT B
Describe the contributions to overall DNP project planning		
Describe the aim/objectives for which Student is taking a leadership role		
Describe contributions to • Writing the DNP project proposal • Proposal presentation • IRB submission • Developing plan for experience • Hours		
Describe the contributions to • Project planning • Project implementation • Project evaluation/data analysis and synthesis		
Describe the contributions to methods of dissemination • Final project paper • Final project poster • Final project presentation		
Other project-related contributions:		
Student signatures:		

IRB, Internal Review Board.

Approved by DNP chair:

Name: _____ **Date:** _____

EXPERIENCE LOG

DATE	COURSE	DESCRIPTION OF EXPERIENCE ACTIVITY	DNP ESSENTIAL DOMAIN	# OF HOURS ANTICIPATED	# OF HOURS COMPLETED	CUMULATIVE HOURS

(continued)

DATE	COURSE	DESCRIPTION OF EXPERIENCE ACTIVITY	DNP ESSENTIAL DOMAIN	# OF HOURS ANTICIPATED	# OF HOURS COMPLETED	CUMULATIVE HOURS

DATE	COURSE	DESCRIPTION OF EXPERIENCE ACTIVITY	DNP ESSENTIAL DOMAIN	# OF HOURS ANTICIPATED	# OF HOURS COMPLETED	CUMULATIVE HOURS

DNP DOMAINS	
1. Knowledge for Nursing Practice	1
2. Person-Centered Care	2
3. Population Health	3
4. Scholarship for the Nursing Discipline	4
5. Quality and Safety	5
6. Interprofessional Partnerships	6
7. Systems-Based Practice	7
8. Informatics and Healthcare Technologies	8
9. Professionalism	9
10. Personal, Professional, and Leadership Development	10

REFERENCES AND RESOURCES

American Association of Colleges of Nursing. (2015). *The doctor of nursing practice: Current issues and clarifying recommendations*. [White paper]. Retrieved from https://www.aacnnursing.org/Portals/42/News/White-Papers/DNP-Implementation-TF-Report-8-15.pdf

American Association of Colleges of Nursing. (2021). *The Essentials: Core competencies for professional nursing education*. [White paper]. Retrieved from https://www.aacnnursing.org/Portals/0/PDFs/Publications/Essentials-2021.pdf

Index

AACN. *See* American Association of Colleges of Nursing (AACN)
advocacy, 286
alternative dissemination, 241
American Association of Colleges of Nursing (AACN), 32, 156, 186, 188, 206, 248
　sub-competencies, 252
　white paper, 276
American Organization for Nurse Leaders (AONL), 260
　leadership competencies, 260
annotation, 139
annual wellness visits (AWVs), 296
AONL. *See* American Organization for Nurse Leaders (AONL)
appraisal of evidence, 144
authoritarian leadership, 14
AWVs. *See* annual wellness visits (AWVs)

basic technology skills, 16
benchmarking, 207
bios, 5
Bloom's taxonomy, 192, 193
body of scholarship, 287
brainstorming, 66, 82
bureaucratic leadership, 15
business cards, 6
business plans, 260
business skills, 259, 260

Centers for Disease Control and Prevention, framework for program evaluation, 284
champion of change, 161
charismatic leadership, 15
chart-audit tools, tips for developing, 208
citation management, 139
clinical practice guidelines (CPGs), 102, 146
Clinical Practice Guidelines We Can Trust, 102
Cochrane Library, 136
cognitive walkthrough, 77

Collaborative Institutional Training Initiative (CITI) Program, 201
committee, 162, 163
communication, 4, 260
community-based projects, 283
competency, 2
competency development, 292
consent, 204
CPGs. *See* clinical practice guidelines (CPGs)
Crossing the Quality Chasm, 42
Cumulative Index to Nursing and Allied Health Literature (CINAHL), 136
curriculum vitae (CV), 9
CV. *See* curriculum vitae (CV)

data analysis, project data and plans for, 209
database, 134, 136
data visualization, 262
date range, 140
democratic leadership, 15
discussion sections, 226
DNP chair, 156
DNP project advisor, 156
Doctor of Nursing Practice (DNP), 36, 45
　engagement
　　in research, 264–265, 266
　　in systematic review, 265, 266
　experience hours, 250, 273
　interprofessional interactions, 273
　versus PhD, 36, 37, 38, 39
　political awareness and engagement, 257
　portfolio, 255
　practice hours, 248
　sources of evidence, 98
Doctor of Nursing Practice (DNP) Project, 24, 102, 186, 276
　advocacy, 286, 288
　aim and objectives, 191
　alternative dissemination, 241
　anticipated findings, 215
　basic technology skills for, 16
　champion of change, 161

　cognitive walkthrough, 77
　Collaborative Institutional Training Initiative (CITI) Program, 201
　common types of, 50–52
　community-based projects, 283
　competencies, 2
　competency development, 292
　data analysis, project data and plans for, 209
　data visualization, 262
　demonstrating value of, 115
　design types of, 49, 50
　developing business skills, 259
　developing writing skills, 18
　discussion sections, 226
　empowerment, 300
　evaluation of outcomes and process, 206
　evidence-based message, 277
　evidence-based projects, 188
　expert commentary, 206
　final academic paper, 231
　global and national problems, 70
　goal of, 49
　historic nursing leadership, 158
　impact and implications, 229
　implementation frameworks, 196
　initial ideas, 68
　initial inquiry and initial search, 93
　Institute for Healthcare Improvement Model for Improvement, 280
　institutional review board, 216
　intended purpose of, 46
　intervention population, 198
　just culture and, 271
　management strategies, 20
　methodology of, 188
　minimum expectations for, 190
　motivational interviewing, 277
　negative or bad results, 298
　networking, 79
　nursing leadership, 292
　oral presentations, 233
　organizations, 222
　organizing your findings, 82
　outcomes, 175
　outline, 118

309

Index

Doctor of Nursing Practice (DNP) Project (cont.)
  participation consent, 204
  perspectives on, 188
  population health, 283, 295
  practice experience, 248
  problem of interest, 92
  problems in healthcare, information and technology, 75
  problem statement, 84, 118, 124
  program evaluation, 295
  project feasibility, 171
  project management, 224
  purpose of, 49
  purpose statement, 177, 178
  recruitment strategies, 198, 199
  repositories, 239
  results, 226
  safety and preparedness skill development, 270
  scholarly posters, 235
  SMART strategy, 192
  social media, 241
  state and local problems, 72
  sub-competencies, 252
  theories, 179
  think beyond education, 194
  timeline, budget, and resources, 212, 213
  topic changes, 289
Doctor of Nursing Practice (DNP) team, 156
  creation, 170
  roles, 164, 165
documentation, 139, 141

EBP. *See* evidence-based practice (EBP)
effective marketing, 259
electronic health records, 98
empowerment, 300
engagement
  in research, 264–265, 266
  in systematic review, 265, 266
The Essentials, 29, 32, 164, 248, 252
evidence, 126
  and data, to document the problem, 98
  appraisal, 144
  pyramid, 128
  reviewing and appraising, 124
  synthesizing, 150
evidence-based message, 277
evidence-based practice (EBP), 41, 186
  steps of, 43
evidence-based projects, 188
evidence table, 149
external factors, 225

Federal Emergency Management Association (FEMA), 270
filtered literature, 126

final academic paper, 231
formal literature review, 128
The Future of Nursing, 26, 27, 29

grey literature, 141
  sources, 142
  types, 142

Health Professions Education, 42
healthcare system, 75
health policy, 104, 105
Health Resources Services Administration (HRSA), 296
Healthy People, 100, 109
Healthy People 2030, 270
historic nursing leadership, 158
human factors, 224

infographics, 262, 263
informatics and healthcare technologies, 254
information and technology, 75
informed consent, 204
initial inquiry and initial search, 93, 97
Institute for Healthcare Improvement (IHI), 41, 107, 188
Institute for Healthcare Improvement (IHI) Model for Improvement, 280
institutional review board (IRB), 186, 204, 216, 280
  application considerations, 216
  planning checklist, 217
integrative review, 128, 129
interprofessional interactions, 273
interprofessional partnerships, 254
intervention population, 198
IRBs. *See* institutional review boards (IRBs)

Jewish Community Center, 285
Joanna Briggs Institute (JBI), 136
just culture, 271

keywords, 139
knowledge, 260
  for nursing practice, 252

Laissez-Faire leadership, 14
leadership, 164, 260, 276
leadership development, 175, 255
leadership style, 14
listicles, 262, 263
literature, 126
  types of, 126
literature review, 129
  and appraisal of, 124
literature searche, 143

management strategies, 20
"MAP-IT" framework, 109
marketing, 259
marketing plans, 261
MEDLINE, 136
mitigation, 270
mobile technology, 98
motivational interviewing (MI), 277

negative or bad results, 298
networking, 79
nursing degree *versus* nursing role, 29
Nursing Doctorate (ND) degrees, 24
nursing leadership, 157, 160, 292
nursing management, 157
nursing practice
  knowledge for, 252
  scholarship for, 253

oral presentations, 233
organizations, 222
  basics of, 113
  impact of problem on, 112
  leadership structure, 112
  mission/vision/values of, 112

participation consent, 204
patient/problem, intervention, comparison, outcome (PICO) question, 131, 134
personal account, 140
personal development, 255
personal health records, 98
personal learning, 14
person-centered care, 253
PhD, 24
  versus Doctor of Nursing Practice, 37, 38, 39
Plan, Do, Study, Act, 280, 281
political awareness and engagement, 257
population health, 253, 283, 295
posters, 235
practice experiences, 250
practice gap, 161
prevention, 270
primary literature, 126
problem of interest, 92
problem statement, 84, 118, 124
professional bio, 5
professional competencies, 4
professional development, 4, 255
professionalism, 254, 260
professional pictures, 5
program evaluation, 295
project factors, 225
project feasibility, 171
project management, 224
project management actions, 224
project methodology, goals for, 187

project planning, 156
project procedures, 224
protection, 270
PsycINFO, 137
public health data, 98
PubMed, 137
purpose statement, 177, 178

QI. *See* quality improvement (QI)
Quadruple Aim, 41, 107
qualitative research, 127
quality and safety, 253
quality improvement (QI), 41, 188, 216, 280
    model for, 43
quantitative research, 127
quantitative studies, 144

recovery, 270
recruitment strategies, 198, 199
reflection, 82
repository, 239
response, 270
results of DNP Project, 227
résumés, 9

review and appraisal
    of evidence, 124
    of literature, 124
RHCs. *See* rural health clinics (RHCs)
rural health clinics (RHCs), 296

scholarship for nursing practice, 253
ScienceDirect, 137
scientific method, 44
Scopus, 137
secondary literature, 126
servant leadership, 15
SMART strategy, 192
social determinants of health, 109
social media, 241
spirit of inquiry, 92, 93
stakeholders, 115
strategic agenda, 100
subject headings, 140
surveys, 208
systematic review, 128, 129, 265
systems-based practice, 165, 254

team, 162, 163
team member, 168
terminal nursing, 26
tertiary literature, 126
To Err Is Human in 1999, *Crossing the Quality Chasm*, 41
time management, 20
topic changes, 289
transformational leadership, 15
Triple Aim, 41, 107

UpToDate, 138

validated instruments, tips for, 207

wearable devices, 98
Web of Science, 138
writing skills, 18

YM-YWHA, 285

project planning, 156
project procedures, 224
promotion, 270
PsycINFO, 129
public health data, 96
PubMed, 137
purpose statement, 122, 125

QI. See quality improvement (QI)
Quadruple Aim, 43, 107
qualitative research, 127
quality and safety, 230
quality improvement (QI), 41, 185, 216, 230
  model for, 13
quantitative research, 127
quantitative studies, 144

recovery, 270
recruitment strategies, 198-199
reflection, 82
repository, 259
response, 270
results of DNP Project, 252
resumes, 9

review and appraisal
  of evidence, 124
  of literature, 124
RHCs. See rural health clinics (RHCs)
rural health clinics (RHCs), 96

scholarship for nursing practice, 235
ScienceDirect, 137
scientific method, 44
Scopus, 129
secondary literature, 26
servant leadership, 15
SMART strategy, 192
social determinants of health, 109
social media, 241
spirit of inquiry, 92, 93
stakeholders, 115
strategic agenda, 100
subject headings, 140
surveys, 208
systematic review, 128, 129
systems-based practice, 165, 205

team, 162, 163
team member, 164
terminal nursing, 26
tertiary literature, 126
The Lexus & Olive in 1909, Crossing the Quality Chasm, 41
time management, 20
topic changes, 288
transformational leadership, 15
Triple Aim, 41, 107

UpToDate, 138

standard intervention, tips for, 292

wearable devices, 95
Web of Science, 138
writing skills, 18

YWCA, 285